first place 4 health

Bible Study Series

make every day your best day

Jeannie Blocher

Published by Gospel Light
Ventura, California, U.S.A.
www.gospellight.com
Printed in the U.S.A.

All Scripture quotations, unless otherwise indicated, are taken from the
Holy Bible, New International Version.® Copyright © 1973, 1978, 1984 by
International Bible Society. Used by permission of Zondervan Publishing
House. All rights reserved.

Other versions used are
NKJV—Scripture taken from the *New King James Version.* Copyright © 1979,
1980, 1982 by Thomas Nelson, Inc. Used by permission. All rights reserved.
KJV—*King James Version.* Authorized King James Version.

© 2012 First Place 4 Health. All rights reserved.

Caution: The information contained in this book is intended to be solely for informational and educational purposes. It is assumed that the First Place 4 Health participant will consult a medical or health professional before beginning this or any other weight-loss or physical fitness program.

It is illegal to copy any part of this document without
permission from First Place 4 Health.

Library of Congress Cataloging-in-Publication Data
Make every day your best day ever.
p. cm. — (First place 4 health Bible study series)
ISBN 978-0-8307-6398-6 (trade paper)
1. Christian life—Biblical teaching—Textbooks 2. Health—Religious aspects—
Christianity—Textbooks.
BS680.C47M335 2012
248.4—dc23
2012001905

Rights for publishing this book outside the U.S.A. or in non-English languages are administered by Gospel Light Worldwide, an international not-for-profit ministry. For additional information, please visit www.glww.org, email info@glww.org, or write to Gospel Light Worldwide, 1957 Eastman Avenue, Ventura, CA 93003, U.S.A.

To order copies of this book and other First Place 4 Health products in bulk quantities, please contact us at 1-800-727-5223. You can also order copies from Gospel Light at 1-800-446-7735.

contents

About the Author 4
Foreword by Carole Lewis 5
Introduction 6

BIBLE STUDIES

Week One: Welcome to *Make Every Day Your Best Day* 8
Week Two: Leave Yesterday Behind 9
Week Three: Let Tomorrow Take Care of Itself 25
Week Four: Have the Right Attitude 39
Week Five: Make Wise Decisions One Day at a Time 53
Week Six: Take Small Steps in the Right Direction 69
Week Seven: Watch Out for the Father of Lies 83
Week Eight: Get Your Spiritual Life in Shape 99
Week Nine: Take Care of Your Physical Health 113
Week Ten: Guard Your Heart and Emotions Daily 129
Week Eleven: Give Your Life Away 145
Week Twelve: Time to Celebrate! 161

ADDITIONAL MATERIALS

Leader Discussion Guide 162
First Place 4 Health Menu Plans 174
First Place 4 Health Member Survey 205
Personal Weight and Measurement Record 207
Weekly Prayer Partner Forms 209
Live It Trackers 231
Let's Count Our Miles! 255
Scripture Memory Verses 257

about the author

Jeannie Blocher is the president of Body & Soul Fitness, an international nonprofit ministry that creates Christ-focused fitness alternatives worldwide. Body & Soul trains qualified instructors to teach a variety of faith-based fitness programs in their local churches and gyms. Jeannie and her husband, Roy, founded the ministry of Body & Soul in 1981. She has been a guest speaker on *Focus on the Family* and *Janet Parshall's America*, and has been featured in *Today's Christian Woman* magazine. Jeannie choreographed and led the workout team on the First Place 4 Health fitness DVD series and has been a speaker at numerous First Place 4 Health events. To find out more about Body & Soul Fitness, visit the ministry website, www.bodyandsoul.org.

foreword

My introduction to Bible study came when I joined First Place in March 1981. I had been attending church since I was a small child, but the extent of my study of the Bible had been reading my Sunday School quarterly on Saturday night. On Sunday morning, I would listen to my Sunday School teacher as she taught God's Word to me. During the worship service, I would listen to our pastor as he taught God's Word to me. Frankly, the idea of digging out the truths of the Bible for myself had never entered my mind.

Perhaps you are right where I was back in 1981. If so, you are in for a blessing you never dreamed possible. As you start studying the truths of the Bible for yourself through the First Place 4 Health Bible studies, you will see God begin to open your understanding of His Word.

Almost every First Place 4 Health member I have talked with about the program says, "The weight loss is wonderful, but the most important thing I have received from my association with First Place 4 Health is learning to study God's Word." The First Place 4 Health Bible studies are designed to be done on a daily basis. As you work through each day's study (which will take 15 to 20 minutes to complete), you will be discovering the deep truths of God's Word. A part of each week's study will also include a Bible memory verse for the week.

There are many in-depth Bible studies on the market. The First Place 4 Health Bible studies are not designed for the purpose of in-depth study, but are designed to be used in conjunction with the rest of the program to bring balance into your life. Our desire is for each member to begin having a personal quiet time with God each day. This time alone with God should include a time of prayer, Bible reading and Bible study. Having a quiet time is a daily discipline that will bring the rich rewards of balance, which is something we all need.

God bless you as you begin this exciting journey toward a balanced life. God will richly bless your efforts to give Him first place in your life. Remember Matthew 6:33: "But seek first his kingdom and his righteousness, and all these things will be given to you as well."

Carole Lewis, First Place 4 Health National Director

introduction

First Place 4 Health is a Christ-centered health program that emphasizes balance in the physical, mental, emotional and spiritual areas of life. The First Place 4 Health program is meant to be a daily process. As we learn to keep Christ first in our lives, we will find that He is the One who satisfies our hunger and our every need.

This Bible study is designed to be used in conjunction with the First Place 4 Health program but can be beneficial for anyone interested in obtaining a balanced lifestyle. The Bible study has been created in a five-day format, with the last two days reserved for reflection on the material studied. Keep in mind that the ultimate goal of studying the Bible is not only for knowledge but also for application and a changed life. Don't feel anxious if you can't seem to find the *correct* answer. Many times, the Word will speak differently to different people, depending on where they are in their walk with God and the season of life they are experiencing. Be prepared to discuss with your fellow First Place 4 Health members what you learned that week through your study.

There are some additional components included with this study that will be helpful as you pursue the goal of giving Christ first place in every area of your life:

- **Group Prayer Request Form:** This form is at the end of each week's study. You can use this to record any special requests that might be given in class.

- **Leader Discussion Guide:** This discussion guide is provided to help the First Place 4 Health leader guide a group through this Bible study. It includes ideas for facilitating a First Place 4 Health class discussion for each week of the Bible study.

- **Two Weeks of Menu Plans with Recipes:** There are 14 days of meals, and all are interchangeable. Each day totals 1,400 to 1,500 calories and includes snacks. Instructions are given for those who need more calories. An accompanying grocery list includes items needed for each week of meals.

- **First Place 4 Health Member Survey:** Fill this out and bring it to your first meeting. This information will help your leader know your interests and talents.

- **Personal Weight and Measurement Record:** Use this form to keep a record of your weight loss. Record any loss or gain on the chart after the weigh-in at each week's meeting.

- **Weekly Prayer Partner Forms:** Fill out this form before class and place it into a basket during the class meeting. After class, you will draw out a prayer request form, and this will be your prayer partner for the week. Try to call or email the person sometime before the next class meeting to encourage that person.

- **Live It Trackers:** Your Live It Tracker is to be completed at home and turned in to your leader at your weekly First Place 4 Health meeting. The Tracker is designed to help you practice mindfulness and stay accountable with regard to your eating and exercise habits. Step-by-step instructions for how to use the Live It Tracker are provided in the *Member's Guide*.

- **Let's Count Our Miles!** A worthy goal we encourage is for you to complete 100 miles of exercise during your 12 weeks in First Place 4 Health. There are many activities listed on pages 255-256 that count toward your goal of 100 miles. When you complete a mile of activity, mark off the box listed on the Hundred Mile Club chart located on the inside of the back cover.

- **Scripture Memory Cards:** These cards have been designed so you can use them while exercising. It is suggested that you punch a hole in the upper left corner and place the cards on a ring. You may want to take the cards in the car or to work so you can practice each week's Scripture memory verse throughout the day.

- **Scripture Memory CD:** All 10 Scripture memory verses have been put to music at an exercise tempo in the CD at the back of this study. Use this CD when exercising or even when you are just driving in your car. The words of Scripture are often easier to memorize when accompanied by music.

Week One

welcome to
Make Every Day Your Best Day

At your first group meeting for this session of First Place 4 Health, you will meet your fellow members, get an overview of your materials and find out what you can expect at weekly meetings. The majority of your class time will be spent learning about the four-sided person concept, the Live It Food Plan, and how change begins from the inside out. You will also have a chance to ask any questions about how to get the most out of First Place 4 Health. If possible, complete the Member Survey on page 205 before your first group meeting. The information that you give will help your leader tailor the next 12 weeks to the needs of the whole group.

Each weekly meeting begins with a weigh-in for members. This will allow you to track your progress over the 12-week session. Your Week One weigh-in/measurement will establish a baseline of comparison so that you can set healthy goals for this session. If you are apprehensive about weighing in every week, talk with your group leader about your concerns. He or she will have some options for you to consider that will make the weigh-in activity encouraging rather than stressful.

The day after your first meeting, begin Week Two of this Bible study. This study is a companion to *Live Life Right Here, Right Now!* by Carole Lewis, so you will want to read that book before beginning. This session, you will focus on spiritual, physical, mental and emotional aspects of your life and how to make wise choices in each area as you make every day your best day. As you open yourself to the truth of Scripture and share your hopes and struggles with the members of your group during the next 12 weeks, you'll find yourself becoming the healthy child of God you are designed to be!

Week Two

leave yesterday behind

SCRIPTURE MEMORY VERSE
Forget the former things; do not dwell on the past.
ISAIAH 43:18

Carpe diem is a Latin phrase that means "seize the day." It can be loosely translated to mean "enjoy, use or make use of this day." When it comes right down to it, don't we often find ourselves "missing the day" instead of seizing it? Too many times we do not use our days well. We find ourselves looking back at the day and wondering where the time went. We realize that we have missed the best that the day had for us, and we ask ourselves, *What did I accomplish today?*

Starting right here, right now, you can make changes in your life so that every day can be your best day. It is our hope and prayer that this study will guide you to embrace life one day at a time, seizing each day and using it wisely in the power of the Holy Spirit. This week, we will explore together how we can let go of the past, seize each day as it comes, and look forward with hope to the future. As you begin, consider the following quote from "The Lifebuilder's Creed" by Dale Witherington:

> Today. This moment. NOW. It is God's gift to me. It is all that I have. Today is what God has entrusted to me. It is all that I have. I will do my best in it. I will demonstrate the best of me in it—my character, giftedness, and abilities—to my family, and friends, clients and associates, I will identify those things that are most important to do Today, and those things I will do until they are

done. And when this day is done I will look back with satisfaction at that which I have accomplished. Then, and only then, will I plan my tomorrow, looking to improve upon Today, with God's help.[1]

Are you ready to make this creed the desire of your heart?

Day 1 — LET GO OF THE PAST

Lord, today I ask for Your supernatural power to leave my past behind and dwell in the present. Allow everything in my past that brings me pain, guilt and sorrow to fade into Your sea of forgetfulness. Amen.

As you begin this First Place 4 Health study and start to memorize Isaiah 43:18, the memory verse for this week, be sure to understand and take to heart the point being made in the verse: As you grow in your relationship with God, He wants you to leave some things behind. He does not want you to dwell on negatives from your past.

Now read Isaiah 43:19. Are you ready for a new thing to spring up in you? Can you sense it coming? Write down your hopes and expectations about the "new thing" that God is going to do in each area of your life—emotionally, spiritually, mentally and physically—as a result of being a part of the First Place 4 Health program.

Emotionally

_____
_____

Spiritually

_____
_____

Mentally

_____
_____
_____

Physically

_____
_____
_____

Have you ever been in a place where it felt as if your life was a "wasteland" (Isaiah 43:19)? Have you felt that "desert" feeling of being desperately thirsty for something better? God promises in this verse to make a way for you to pass through and out of that desert—a way for you to find the refreshing streams He has for you. Read John 4:11-14. Why will people who drink the water that Jesus provides never be thirsty (see verse 14)?

_____
_____
_____
_____

Read John 7:37-38. How do we obtain the "streams of living water" (see verse 38)?

_____
_____
_____
_____

Right now, go get a glass of water. Drink it slowly and imagine the Lord bringing cool, fresh water into the desert parts of your life. Think of a stream gushing into the wasteland parts of your life, bringing new hope. Each day this week, start your day with a glass of water and focus on God and His plan to refresh you and give you living water. Review the memory verse as you drink. Create this new habit and get excited about the new thing that God is doing in your life! Now read Ezekiel 36:26. What is God giving you, and what is He removing from you?

What will this look like in your life?

Read 2 Corinthians 5:17. What does "in Christ" mean?

When we are "in Christ," what do we become?

Take time right now to think about and write down things on which you must no longer dwell (hurts you've suffered and never forgiven, negative words you've heard about yourself or negative thoughts you've had about yourself, former attempts at weight loss, and so forth). Add to this list any other things God brings to your mind.

When the old has gone, the new comes. Think about the "new creation" that you want to be and how your lifestyle will change as a result. What will be different emotionally, spiritually, mentally and physically? Start to write down these things now in your journal, and keep working all week on the changes that you want to see so that at the end of the week you will have a vision statement of the new you!

Thank You, Lord, that You have forgotten my past. Help me to leave it behind so that I can seize each today and live it to Your glory. Amen.

SEIZE THE DAY AND REJOICE

Day 2

Lord, guide me to rejoice in today because You have made it. Help me to give the sacrifice of praise to You, even in difficult circumstances. Amen.

As we begin to experience newness in our lives, joy grows in our hearts. It may start as a small trickle of hope, but it can bubble up into daily rejoicing if we nurture it. Read Psalm 118:24. What does "rejoice and be glad in [each day]" mean?

___

Using a scale of 1 to 10—with 10 being the easiest—how easy would you find it to live out this verse each day? Why?

___

Read Isaiah 43:20-21, which provides more of the context of our memory verse. Why should we rejoice?

___

What is your natural response when someone gives you something?

_____
_____
_____
_____

What are five things that God has given you?

1. _____
2. _____
3. _____
4. _____
5. _____

A final word of encouragement is found in Isaiah 44:2-4. List two things that God will do for you because He has chosen you.

1. _____
2. _____

Think of a difficult situation you've faced recently. If at that time you gave a sacrifice of praise, what happened? If you didn't, how do you think a sacrifice of praise would have helped?

_____
_____
_____
_____

Lord, help me to praise You in all circumstances—when the sun is shining and in the midst of the storms of life. I know I can grow in this area, and I will not be afraid. Amen.

LIVE FREE FROM GUILT — Day 3

Lord, I am tired of fighting the guilt of my past. Teach me how to leave this behind and live life in the present, serving You with a heart that is free. Amen.

One thing that often keeps us from rejoicing in each day and making each day our best is the guilt from our pasts that hovers over us. Today, let's explore what the Bible has to say about why we should leave the guilt behind us. Read Psalm 38:1-8. What was causing David's problem (see verses 3-4)?

How did David feel (see verses 5-8)?

According to what David wrote in Psalm 32, how are our guilty consciences cleansed (see verse 5)?

What do we have because we believe in Jesus (see Ephesians 1:7)?

Read Ephesians 2:4-8. What do we have to do to earn God's saving grace?

_____
_____
_____

Read Micah 7:18-20. Even if we feel as if God will never forgive our sins or free us from the guilt we feel, why should we still be encouraged to live free from guilt (see verse 18)?

_____
_____
_____

What will God do with our sins (see verse 19)?

_____
_____
_____

Father, thank You for forgiving my sins. I know it is because of Your loving mercy that I can leave the guilt of my past behind. My hope is in You alone.

Day 4: TRUST OUR UNCHANGEABLE GOD

Lord, it is so easy for me to get stuck in yesterday. Help me to trust You more today and have hope for tomorrow. Guide me to leave my past behind as I focus on You. Amen.

As we move forward to leave our past behind, live in the present and look forward to tomorrow, we gain hope by focusing on God. We can count on Him to always be with us. Read Malachi 3:6. What did the Lord say about Himself?

_____
_____
_____

Read Hebrews 13:8. What did the writer of Hebrews say about Jesus?

Read James 1:17. How did James describe God?

How is all of creation different from God?

Read Proverbs 3:5-8. What five things are we encouraged to do?

1.
2.
3.
4.
5.

What will God do in return (see verses 6,8)?

Lord, draw me closer and closer to You as my trust in You grows. Strengthen me so that I will keep my eyes on You. Help me to remember that You never change and that You will always be with me. Amen.

Day 5 — LOOK FORWARD TO THE FUTURE

Heavenly Father, I know that You will use everything that happens in my life for my good. Help me to remember this when I am struggling with my circumstances. Amen.

As we learn how to leave the past behind and rejoice in today, we also need to see that tomorrow is part of God's plan. God works things together for our good at *all* times, and this includes the future. Read Romans 8:28. What does "the good" mean in the context of this verse?

For whom does God do this?

What does "called according to his purpose" mean (see also Ephesians 3:11)?

That phrase, "God works for the good of those who love him," rolls off the tongue so easily, but when life brings storms, our troubles usually shake our confidence and make us question what's going on. Read Isaiah 55:8-9. What are God's thoughts and ways like?

Read Psalm 145:3. How did David describe God's greatness?

Read Psalm 139:2,17. How do our thoughts compare to God's?

How do you feel about the fact that God's thoughts and ways are beyond your capability to understand them? Does that give you comfort or bring uncertainty? Why?

Briefly describe a time when God was working something for your good, but at the time it didn't really feel good. How do you now see that God was at work for your good, even when you had no understanding of that at the time?

Lord, I know You desire to work all things together for good in my life. Help me to seek You every day and listen as You speak Your thoughts to me. Amen.

Day 6

REFLECTION AND APPLICATION

Dear Lord, help me to leave behind the "former things" in my life that weigh me down and hold me back. Help me to seek the "new thing" that You are doing in me. Amen.

The Dead Sea is water, but it is different from what most of us think of when we hear the word "sea." When you step into it, you have to be careful to wear beach or water shoes so that you don't hurt your feet stepping on the clumps of salt crystals that form on the bottom. Once you're in the water, you marvel at how you are so buoyant that you float to the top in an instant. People grab handfuls of the mud from the bottom and smear it on their skin for a beauty treatment. But no one considers drinking it. This water is loaded with so much salt that it would never be refreshing. Animals can't drink it either; in fact, no animal can live *in* it. There is a reason that it is called the Dead Sea!

In some ways, your former life is like the water in the Dead Sea. It is not life-giving. Remember the glass of water you drank on the first day of this study? Have you made it a habit yet to drink water every day? Here are some practical tips for adding water to your life. See how many things you can check off today and add to your list of healthy habits.

- ☐ Pull out your favorite water bottle, or treat yourself to a new water bottle or insulated cup. Pick a fun color and style and a size that you can carry in your purse or bag when you go out. Fill it each night and chill it in the refrigerator if you like.

- ☐ When you first wake up, take a big drink of this water you have prepared and start your day with the refreshing feeling that reminds you that a "new thing" is springing up in your life!

- ☐ Review your Scripture memory verse for the week as you drink your first glass of water for the day.

- ☐ After breakfast, fill your water bottle again. Take it with you if you are going out, or, if you are staying home, put it on a coaster on your desk or countertop where you will have easy access to it throughout your morning. Drink water from your bottle often throughout the day, and each time you do, make it a time of connecting to God in a brief prayer. He is the giver of living water! (Read the story in John 4.)

- ☐ Omit sugary drinks and focus on water being your main drink all day long. There is an amazing phenomenon that happens: When you drink water, you actually crave more water!

Review this list every day and make drinking water one of your new healthy habits. The bonus is that you will even save money as you focus on water as one of your healthy choices!

Thank You, Lord Jesus, that You give living water to each one of us every day. Help me to create this new healthy habit of drinking water, starting this week. Amen.

REFLECTION AND APPLICATION — Day 7

Lord, give me a new vision for who I can be as Your child. Help me to write my vision for a new me, the person You created me to be. Amen.

On Day 1, you were asked to start jotting down ideas about the new creation you want to be and how your lifestyle will change as a result. Today, write your detailed personal vision statement. Write it in the first person and in present tense (not future tense). Describe what you look like, how you feel and what your attitude about life is. Describe how you order your day to prioritize health and fitness in all areas of your life: emotionally, mentally, physically and spiritually.

Include what you do during the day and the people with whom you spend your time. Describe how you connect with God each day and how you serve God in your world. Basically, imagine your ideal life so you can envision the new thing that God is doing in you as you leave the former things behind. You may be able to just start writing and the thoughts will flow, or you may feel more comfortable using the guided thoughts below:

When I wake up, my first thoughts are about _____

_____

_____

I start my day spiritually by _____

_____

_____

When I pray, I always include _____

_____

_____

I begin my healthy eating habits by _____

_____

_____

My exercise choice for the day is _____

_____

_____

My morning is filled by _____

_____

_____

I like to do things with _____

_____

_____

My attitude for the day is _____

_____

_____

For lunch I like _____

_____

_____

My afternoon includes _____

_____

_____

I make time to serve God by _____

_____

_____

My evening meal is _____

_____

_____

After dinner I enjoy _____

_____

_____

Before going to sleep, I connect with God by _____

_____

_____

Heavenly Father, thank You for giving me a vision of how my life can change as a result of seeking You through this study. Help me to make wise choices each day so I can move closer to this vision of health that You have given me. Amen.

Note
1. Dale Witherington, "The Lifebuilder's Creed," quoted in John Maxwell, *Today Matters: 12 Daily Practices to Guarantee Tomorrow's Success* (New York: Time Warner Book Group, 2004), pp. 13-14.

Group Prayer Requests

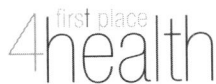

Today's Date: _____

Name	Request

Results

Week Three

let tomorrow take care of itself

SCRIPTURE MEMORY VERSE
Therefore do not worry about tomorrow, for tomorrow will worry about itself. Each day has enough trouble of its own.
MATTHEW 6:34

Reading this verse can make us think about what we hear on our local news station. We want to be aware of what is going on in the world, but sometimes we have to turn the television off or shut down the Internet site and just let "tomorrow . . . worry about itself," because today "has enough trouble of its own." When we insulate ourselves against things in life that tend to cause us to worry unnecessarily, we protect ourselves from worry itself.

A wise woman once said, "Enjoy each season of your life. Don't miss the present because of worry over the future. Life is what happens right here, right now." This same idea is reflected in Scripture in many ways, such as in this week's memory verse and in Ecclesiastes 3:1, where Solomon writes, "There is a time for everything, and a season for every activity under heaven."

This week, we will explore how we can cast our cares on God, letting go of worry about tomorrow and leaving our days in His capable hands. We will also examine how we can live an abundant life each and every day of our lives. We have been given every reason to trust in God and be comforted by His vigilant care, and we should be overjoyed that God is in control of everything, instead of us!

Day 1

GIVE GOD YOUR WORRIES

Lord, help me to give my worries to You daily. Help me to let go of them and trust You to take care of them. Amen.

God assures us in His Word that we can give all of our cares and worries to Him. As difficult as it may be for us to imagine, God can handle the things that cause us stress a lot better than we can. Read Psalm 55:22. What did David say that we should do with our cares?

_____
_____
_____
_____

Write your own definition of the word "cares." When you cast your cares on the Lord, what are you handing over to Him?

_____
_____
_____
_____

Can you picture yourself holding all of your cares in your arms and then throwing them up in the air and watching them disappear into the heavenlies for God to take care of them? Picture yourself doing this. What will God do when we cast our cares on Him?

_____
_____
_____

According to 1 Peter 5:7, why should we give God our anxieties?

_____
_____
_____

Read Matthew 6:25-32. What things did Jesus say not to worry about?

What can worry not do (see verse 27)? How does this affect your thoughts about worrying?

Read Psalm 139:23-24. What are four things that David asked God to do?

1.
2.
3.
4.

If you were to ask God to search and examine your heart, what would He find there? A lot of worries? Anything offensive? Anything you would try to hide? Explain.

Lord, I want You to search me and know my heart. I know that You are aware of my anxious thoughts. Help me to cast all of them on You. Amen.

Day 2 — EXCHANGE WORRIES FOR TRUST

Lord, help me to exchange my worries for trust in You. I thank You ahead of time for helping me to grow in this area. Amen.

It's easy for us to say, "I'll give all my worries to God and won't worry," but it's difficult for our minds to instantly cut off our concerns. Our thoughts want to return to the things that bother us. So what do we do? We *exchange* the worrisome thoughts for something else: trust in God. Look up Isaiah 30:15. What happens when we trust God?

According to Isaiah 26:3, what else will God do when we trust Him?

Read Psalm 56:3-4. What is the antidote for fear?

Because of his trust in God, of whom was David not afraid?

Turn to Psalm 20:7. What are some of the "chariots and horses" that people trust in the world today?

According to Psalm 9:10, why can God be trusted?

What are a few specific steps you can take that will guide you to think first about trusting in God when you experience any worrisome situation?

Dear Lord, help me to turn to You when I start to worry and when I am afraid. I trust You with my time, my loved ones, my finances and my life. Amen.

LIVE AN ABUNDANT LIFE EVERY DAY

Day 3

Lord, help me to focus on living one day at a time, enjoying each day as it comes and living life to its fullest. Amen.

We need to change our paradigm in order to focus on one day at a time. We are so used to planning for the future and thinking about tomorrow that many of us are missing out on today. The reality is that life *is* today. What happens in the here and now *is* life. And God wants it to be a full life! Read John 10:10. For what reason did Jesus say He came to this world? What did He mean by this?

What does "having life to the full" look like for you?

Turn to Philippians 4:5-9. After exhorting us to not be anxious, what did Paul encourage us to do, and in what manner (see verse 6)?

Why do you think it is important not only to do this but also to do it in this manner?

Why is presenting our requests before God an important habit for us to develop?

What will happen as a result (see verse 7)?

How have you experienced this blessing in your life?

What should be the focus of our daily thoughts (see verse 8)?

How will thinking about such things influence our words and actions?

Think of at least one specific way you can put into practice what you have learned in today's study. Then do it—and strive to put it into practice *every* day!

Heavenly Father, thank You for reminding me of the value of focusing on living well. Help me to pursue habits that will turn my heart away from worry and toward You. Thank You for the peace that transcends understanding that You promise. Amen.

RECOGNIZE THAT GOD IS IN CONTROL

Day 4

Lord, You know I like to know what's coming next. Help me to understand that the only thing that matters is that You are in control. Thank You for guiding my life. Amen.

Living without knowing the timeline of everything and without being able to control every event can be difficult. We like to know what is coming next—and precisely when it will happen. We like answers and order. But we are not in control. Only God is. Once we realize this, our trust in Him will grow stronger and stronger, and our worries will lessen. Read Acts 1:7-8. What did Jesus tell His disciples about the timeline for what was going to come to pass?

Jesus abruptly changed the subject of this conversation. What did He consider to be more important for them to know?

Read Acts 2:4. What happened when the Holy Spirit came to the disciples? How did they show that they were in the power of, or being controlled by, the Holy Spirit?

Do you feel as if the Holy Spirit is at work in you and through you, just as it was for the disciples (note that this need not be displayed by your speaking in different languages!)? Briefly describe a time when you felt the leading of the Holy Spirit.

According to Job 12:9-10, what does God hold in His hand?

According to Proverbs 16:9 and 19:21, what does God determine for us?

When we obey God, what does He do for us as we walk with Him (see Psalm 37:23-24)?

_____
_____
_____

Read Deuteronomy 32:4. Why is it better that God is in control rather than us?

_____
_____
_____

Lord, help me to recognize that You are not only the Creator of all things but also the controller of all things. My heart's desire is to leave my future in Your hands and live with joy today. Amen.

BE COMFORTED BY GOD'S VIGILANT CARE

Day 5

Dear heavenly Father, thank You for watching over me every day, every hour, every minute. I know I am safe in Your loving care. Amen.

The Bible makes it clear that God watches over His creation—*all* of His creation. The fact that God is always watching over us should reassure us of His loving care, no matter what happens. Remember what David wrote: "In God I trust; I will not be afraid. What can mortal man do to me?" (Psalm 56:4). Read the following verses. Next to each verse, write who or what God watches over:

Psalm 33:18 _____

Psalm 127:1 _____

Psalm 145:20 _____

Psalm 146:9 (three are mentioned) _____
_____
_____

Read Psalm 121. Note how many times it mentions that God is watching over us. What are at least three different things that God does for us as He watches over us?

1. _____
2. _____
3. _____

When does God take His eyes off of us (see verses 3-4)?

_____
_____
_____

Read Genesis 28:10-15. Jacob left his parents and brother and went to live with Laban. Along the way, he stopped one night to sleep and had an unusual dream. Why did Jacob need reassurance at this time? (If you're not familiar with the story of Esau and Jacob, read Genesis 25:19-34; 27.)

_____
_____
_____

What promises did God make to Jacob (see verses 13,15)?

_____
_____
_____

The promise in verse 15 is for all of us. It is a reaffirmation that God is watching over us wherever we go. Read Jeremiah 31:10. To what is God compared, and why is this a good description?

_____
_____
_____

Turn to John 10:11-18. What did Jesus call Himself? What reasons did He give for calling Himself this?

_____
_____
_____
_____

Briefly describe a time when you felt God's eyes watching over you. What effect did it have on you and your actions?

_____
_____
_____
_____

Think of several people that you know who need a special touch from God this week. Take time to pray specifically for God to watch over them closely.

Dear Lord, I am grateful that You are there for me in all circumstances. Just as You reassured Jacob, reassure me and stay close to me. Amen.

REFLECTION AND APPLICATION

Day 6

Dear Lord, I need Your help one day at a time and one decision at a time. I want to continue to move away from worry and toward trust in You. Amen.

Most of us probably know that it is impossible for us to decide all at once to stop worrying and let tomorrow take care of itself. We cannot do it in a day, or even in a week. It is a process. With this in mind, when a worry enters your mind and heart today, look back at the approaches we covered this week and try one so that you can exchange your worry for trust. Next, make a conscious decision to trust God to take care of that specific worry. Do this for the rest of the worries you encounter. At the end of today, stop and assess your progress.

What worked? What didn't work?

_____
_____
_____
_____

Did you make any improvement in how you handled worry? If not, what got in the way of you doing this?

_____
_____
_____
_____

What can you do to improve so that you worry less and trust God more tomorrow?

_____
_____
_____
_____

Thank You, Lord, for helping me make one worry-to-trust decision at a time, each and every day. Guide me away from worry and toward more trust in You. Amen.

Day 7 — REFLECTION AND APPLICATION

Lord, You are the air I breathe. I'm lost without You. Help me to breathe You in each day and breathe out my worries and cares. Amen.

Today, it's time to start a practical stress-reducing habit: deep breathing! This is not only something that is good for you when you are doing certain exercises, but it is also a daily habit that will help to de-stress your life. In her book *Accidentally Overweight: Solve Your Weight Loss Puzzle*,

Dr. Libby Weaver says that one of the positive benefits to the physical discipline of diaphragmatic breathing is that it will help to lower the stress level in your life.[1]

With this is mind, start your day with 10 deep breaths. (Starting tomorrow, do the 10 deep breaths before getting out of bed. For today, do the breaths now.) Breathe in through your nose and let your breath out slowly through pursed lips. Allow your stomach to expand. This is not shallow chest breathing, so don't rush it. And this is only the beginning. At any time during the day when you feel stressed or start to worry, stop and breathe—just breathe!

While you are taking your 10 deep breaths, practice your memory verse or say a prayer. Or you could listen to the worship song "Breathe" by Michael W. Smith while you enjoy several minutes of wonderful reflective breathing. It's pretty hard to worry when you are focused on the Lord and doing relaxing breathing techniques!

Heavenly Father, thank You for giving me resources to use so that I can focus on You and not on my worries. Help me to be faithful to make the changes in my life that are needed. I love You. Amen.

Note
1. Libby Weaver, *Accidentally Overweight: Solve Your Weight Loss Puzzle* (New Zealand: Little Green Frog Publishing Ltd., 2010).

Group Prayer Requests

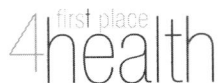

Today's Date: _____

Name	Request

Results

_____
_____
_____
_____
_____

Week Four

have the right attitude

SCRIPTURE MEMORY VERSE
But I trust in you, O LORD; I say, "You are my God." My times are in your hands.
PSALM 31:14-15

Attitude. We hear a lot today about people who have an attitude. We don't want our teenagers to have an attitude. We don't like it when a clerk in a store where we are shopping has an attitude. We certainly don't want to see someone driving recklessly because they have an attitude. But what about our own attitude? We need to take an honest look at how our attitude affects our lives today and every day. And we need to be willing to make an attitude adjustment as needed at any given moment—in God's power.

Today, we will look at the types of attitudes we have and how we can change them through the renewal of our minds. We will learn that, as believers, our attitude should always be one of thankfulness, no matter what is our situation or our circumstance. Our God is a great God who has given us many reasons to rejoice and be thankful. We just need to make an attitude adjustment so we have the right attitude today and every day.

RENEW YOUR MIND

Day 1

Lord, help me to be aware of my attitude so I can relate to people in my life as a reflection of Your love each and every day. Amen.

David almost always had the right attitude. Yes, only "almost"—he *was* human, so he did make a few mistakes! David's psalms, though, do reflect the attitude we should have. Read Psalm 31:9-20, the context of our memory verse for the week. Why did David call on God (see verses 9-13)?

In spite of his troubles, what was David's attitude (see verses 14-15)?

Why did David have this attitude (see verses 19-20)?

Read Philippians 4:11-13. What is the key attitude that Paul says that he learned (see verses 11-12)?

Why was Paul able to have this attitude (see verse 13)?

When we are working on our attitude, there is a process through which we must go. Read Romans 12:1-2. What are we to offer to God, and how do we do that?

What are some of the patterns (beliefs or practices) of this world to which we should no longer conform?

_____
_____
_____

How does what you think about affect your attitude?

_____
_____
_____

What are a few specific steps that you can take to renew your mind so that it aligns more closely to what God wants?

_____
_____
_____

Heavenly Father, I want to be honest about my own attitude. Forgive me for any wrong attitudes I have shown in the past, and guide me to transform and renew my mind so I can have an attitude that honors You today and every day.

NURTURE HOPE — Day 2

Lord, I want to be a person who is living each day with hope, trusting You so I never despair. I can do this with Your help. You are my hope, O God. Amen.

One of the many wonderful things about God is that He gives us hope so that no matter what our circumstances are, we can confidently look forward to what He has promised. We *expect* that He will deliver on His promises. Read Romans 15:13. What is the relationship between God and hope?

_____
_____
_____

Read Psalm 42. Why is the psalmist upset (see verses 9-10)?

What does the psalmist tell his soul to do (see verses 5-6,11)?

What does the psalmist say about God's presence in the midst of his crisis? Is God ever absent (see verse 8)? ?

Why do you think praising God is connected to hope in Him?

According to Psalm 62:5 and Isaiah 40:31, what happens to those who hope in God?

Read Psalm 147:11. In what attribute of God does this verse say we should specifically place our hope?

According to Romans 12:12, what are we urged to do as we hope?

_____
_____
_____

Dear Lord, You give me rest and renew my strength as I hope in You. Your love never fails. Help me to always be joyful in hope and to praise You no matter what circumstances in life come my way. Amen.

GIVE YOURSELF A BREAK — Day 3

Lord, help me to be kind to myself and give myself room to grow and change. Remove negative thought patterns from my mind and give me a new mindset about myself. Amen.

Sometimes, the hardest attitudes to change are the ones we have about ourselves. Most people tend to be hard on themselves and expect more from themselves than anyone else. Most people also find forgiving themselves difficult, if not impossible. But that's not what God wants of us. Read Psalm 139:1-16. What does God know about us?

_____
_____
_____

According to Romans 8:38-39, what is God's attitude regarding us?

_____
_____
_____

Turn to Romans 8:1-2. What does *not* happen to those who believe in Jesus as their Savior?

_____
_____
_____

Jesus had an interesting encounter in Mark 9:14-29 that reveals how our beliefs about ourselves affect our attitudes (the same event is also related in Matthew 17:14-20 and Luke 9:37-43). One day, a man who had a son afflicted by an evil spirit approached Jesus for help. The evil spirit within the boy often made him mute and suffer from seizures, and his father wanted Jesus to heal his son. However, what about the man's words tells us that he wasn't totally sure Jesus could help the boy (see verses 22-23)?

What did Jesus say about what belief can do (see verse 23)?

What did the father have to say about his belief (see verse 24)? How is our belief often like the father's?

What did Jesus do for the boy (see verses 25-27)?

What was the reason Jesus gave for the disciples' inability to help the boy (see verse 29)?

Why is prayer an excellent way to bolster belief?

_____
_____
_____
_____

Have you ever felt an attitude of condemnation toward yourself? In light of God's love for you, will you commit to let the condemnation go and strive for an attitude of acceptance toward yourself? Believe that with God anything is possible, and He will help you. Stop and pray for the Lord to empower you to move in this direction. Become a prayer warrior in the area of belief—both for yourself and for others—and be prepared to see some impossible things turn into the possible! Start today!

Heavenly Father, I do believe in myself, but I also need You to help my unbelief. Guide me to be the prayer warrior I need to be so that I can see the impossible become possible in my life. Amen.

HAVE COMPASSION TOWARD OTHERS

Day 4

Jesus, give me a heart to understand others. Guide my eyes to see their needs. I want to have an attitude of compassion toward everyone, as You did. Amen.

One of the most impressive characteristics of Jesus was His constant attitude of compassion toward all the people with whom He came into contact. It is this attitude that we all should have toward others. Read Matthew 9:35-36. What was Jesus busy doing, and why?

_____
_____
_____
_____

Turn to Matthew 14:13-21. At one point, Jesus went by boat to be alone for a while, but the crowds followed Him. Even though He had planned to be by Himself, what did He do when He got off the boat, and why (see verses 13-14)?

What did Jesus tell His disciples to do (see verse 16)?

What problem did the disciples have with Jesus' instruction, and how did Jesus solve the issue (see verses 17-21)?

Read Matthew 15:29-39 (see also Mark 8:1-10). What did Jesus do for the people, and why (see verses 30,32)?

Read Matthew 16:5-12. What warning did Jesus give to the disciples? What was their response (see verses 6-7)?

Read Colossians 3:12-14. With what attitudes should we "clothe" ourselves (verse 12)?

Which of these attitudes is the easiest for you? Which is the hardest?

What are some of the things we need to do in order to show off our new "clothes" (see verses 13-14)?

According to Ephesians 4:29-32, what are some additional things we need to do?

Think about how your manner of speaking and the actual words you use reflect your attitude. Speak words of compassion and encouragement to everyone with whom you come into contact this week—and then make such words a daily habit!

> *Lord, help me to grow in compassion each and every day.*
> *Guide me to speak only words that build up people. Amen.*

Day 5

REJOICE AND BE THANKFUL

Heavenly Father, thank You for all You are doing in my life. Help me to be a joy-filled, thankful person. With Your help, I can grow in this area. Amen.

Although the happiness people feel at any given moment usually depends on their circumstances, believers don't have such a limit. Our happiness is constant because of what Jesus did for us, and for that we should always rejoice and be thankful. Start today by reading 1 Thessalonians 5:16-18. What three key things are we encouraged to do?

1. _____
2. _____
3. _____

What is the reason for doing these things (see verse 18)?

_____
_____
_____

Psalm 100 is a great psalm of rejoicing and thankfulness, with the thoughts about joy flowing right into thoughts about giving thanks. For what attributes of God is the psalmist thankful (see verses 3,5)?

_____
_____
_____

Included in the book of 1 Chronicles is a wonderful song of rejoicing and thankfulness by King David. Read 1 Chronicles 16:8-36. Although David urged us to do many things, what five things stand out for you?

1. _____
2. _____
3. _____

4. _____
5. _____

Read Romans 5:3-5. Why did Paul say we should rejoice and be thankful, even when we have problems or troubling circumstances?

_____
_____
_____

According to Philippians 4:4, when should we rejoice?

_____
_____
_____

How are rejoicing and thankfulness related? Why should these two attitudes be at the center of our lives?

_____
_____
_____

Heavenly Father, I give thanks to You! I want to make known what You have done and tell of Your wonderful acts. My heart is glad as I seek Your face. I am looking to You and Your strength. Amen.

REFLECTION AND APPLICATION

Day 6

Dear Lord, I want to put into action things that will help me have a better attitude in all areas of my life. Bring to my mind the things You want me to focus on. Help me to take action to make positive changes in my lifestyle, starting today. Amen.

Today, go back to each of the lessons for this week and choose one nugget of truth that was especially helpful to you. Write it down, and then write the action that you plan to take to make that truth a part of your life—what change you need to make so that what you learned becomes part of your everyday "wardrobe."

Day	Nugget of truth	Action plan
1		
2		
3		
4		
5		

Start today to put each of your plans of action into place, and then watch to see God at work in your life!

Thank You, Lord, that You care about me and love me. I need You to be my strength as I make Your truths part of my life so every day is my best day.

Day 7

REFLECTION AND APPLICATION

Lord, today I ask that You draw near to me as I seek You to know how to move forward. Guide me to choose healthy habits so that I have the right attitude at all times. Amen.

As we discussed this week, a big part of having a healthy attitude is to continually develop a lifestyle of praise and worship for our heavenly

Father. Today, stop right where you are and list below the first 10 things that come to mind for which you are thankful to God for bringing into your life. Note that these can be big or small, because even little things will affect your attitude.

1. _____
2. _____
3. _____
4. _____
5. _____
6. _____
7. _____
8. _____
9. _____
10. _____

Keep adding to this "thankfulness list" by writing down a few items each day for which you are thankful. When you pray, include thanks for these things to God, and rejoice in His many wonderful attributes. Pray prayers of thankfulness the moment that you wake up in the morning and the moment you go to bed at night. Be creative and think of things that happened during the day for which you can be thankful and rejoice in God (such as expressing thanks and joy that God has provided you with enough money to pay for the food on your grocery list). Spend time in God's presence and let Him bring things to your mind that He does not want you to miss!

Dear Lord, today I pray that You will help me to change my life habits and take the time to connect with You on a daily basis. Please help me to see all of the blessings that You bring to me each day and to be intentional about expressing my worship and praise to You. Help me to sit still so that I can hear Your voice above the noise of life. I love You, God. Amen.

Group Prayer Requests

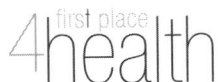

Today's Date: _____

Name	Request

Results

Week Five

make wise decisions one day at a time

SCRIPTURE MEMORY VERSE
*The fear of the LORD is the beginning of wisdom;
all who follow his precepts have good understanding.*
PSALM 111:10

Our decisions shape our lives. Each decision we make carries responsibilities and natural consequences with it. In fact, nothing happens without a reaction of some sort, even though it might not be evident to us at first. For this reason, every decision we make is important, and the best way to make decisions is with wisdom—godly wisdom.

A good definition of wisdom is this: "the ability to discern or judge what is true, right and lasting." That is an accurate depiction of godly wisdom. Another definition says simply that wisdom is "knowing and doing God's will." One thing is for sure: True wisdom is the path to making wise decisions in order to make every day our best day.

What's especially *fortunate* for us is that God can give us wisdom to make right decisions. We just have to ask Him for that wisdom. And, of course, we have God's Word to consult about matters. What's *unfortunate* is that all too often we try to make decisions on our own. We think we already have all the answers, so we certainly don't need to consult God or what He has to say in the Bible about our situation.

However, there is a big difference between earthly wisdom and the eternal view of things. When we learn the difference between what we think we know and what God actually knows, we will have godly wisdom to make the right decision.

Day 1

WISDOM VERSUS UNDERSTANDING

Lord, help me to always seek You before making decisions, knowing that You will guide me to make wise choices every day of my life. Amen.

When most people hear the word "wisdom," they think of facts and figures, information learned from books or knowledgeable people. But true wisdom is from God and begins with reverential fear of our Father Creator. Our memory verse, Psalm 111:10, tells us something vital about wisdom. Where does wisdom begin?

_____

_____

_____

What is the difference between fear, as in being scared, and "fear of the Lord"?

_____

_____

_____

As one writer notes, "Fearing God means approaching Him both as a Father (with boldness and without being afraid of Him) and as the Most High One (with deepest respect)."[1] When we approach God with this appropriate kind of fear, we can be assured that He will give us wisdom to make wise daily decisions. According to the following verses, what are the benefits of being a person who lives with a healthy fear of the Lord?

Scripture	Benefits
Ps. 34:9	
Ps. 85:9	
Ps. 103:17	(1)
	(2)

Scripture	Benefits
Ps. 128:1-4	(1)
	(2)
	(3)
	(4)
Ps. 145:19	(1)
	(2)

There is one more part to our memory verse. When we follow God's commands, we will have good understanding. According to Job 28:28, what is understanding?

_____

_____

_____

Turn to Proverbs 9:10. According to this proverb, what is understanding?

_____

_____

_____

Look at the last part of our memory verse. How do we get understanding?

_____

_____

_____

One of the definitions of "understanding" is "the power of comprehending."[2] Today, when we understand something, we say, "I get it." God wants us to "get it." He wants us to understand Him and His commands. We can do just that when we seek His wisdom. How should knowing that the fear of the Lord is the beginning of wisdom and that understanding is gained by following God's laws affect the decisions we make?

___

Lord, I need both wisdom and understanding. I come boldly before You, with the deepest respect for Your awesome power, and ask for Your help to understand and put into practice Your commands. Amen.

Day 2: EARTHLY WISDOM VERSUS HEAVENLY WISDOM

Dear God, sometimes I feel overwhelmed by the decisions I need to make every day. Guide me to seek You for the decisions that are the best for me and for all the people I love and care about. Amen.

Earthly wisdom and heavenly wisdom are not the same things, nor do they aim for the same goals. Whereas seekers of earthly wisdom hope to gain knowledge and information (often for unscrupulous purposes), seekers of heavenly wisdom hope to gain insight into God and how to win people for God's kingdom. To what do a lot of people in the world turn when they need to "get wisdom"?

___

Read James 1:5-8. What should we do when we feel that we lack wisdom? What sort of response should we expect (see verse 5)?

___

What should our attitude be when we ask (see verses 6-8)?

Go to James 3:13-18. How does a person show that he or she is wise and understanding (see verse 13)?

What are the attributes of earthly wisdom (see verses 14-16)?

What are the attributes of heavenly wisdom (see verses 17-18)?

Read Daniel 12:3. What does this verse say about those who are wise?

What do wise people lead others toward?

Daniel is a great example of a young man who made wise decisions. He stayed true to God. He lived a life that was focused, trusting in God. He was not swayed by peer pressure or tempted by worldly fame or power. His life did shine like the stars!

> *Lord, help me to grow in wisdom so I can be like Daniel, shining like a star in the universe, leading others to righteousness. I desire to be a good decision maker. I trust in You to help me move in that direction, one day at a time.*

Day 3 — WISE DECISIONS VERSUS UNWISE DECISIONS

> *Lord, I know that You are leading me to make wise decisions every day. Help me to learn as I go, walking closely with You and taking to heart the truth in Your Word. Amen.*

King Solomon is an example of a man who made many wise decisions and some very unwise ones, and we can learn from what he did. We can determine to make wise decisions throughout our lives and not to stray from what we know is right. Read 1 Kings 3:4-15. For what did Solomon ask God? What was God's response (see verses 9-14)?

What condition did God put on Solomon for a long life (see verse 14)?

How did Solomon respond (see verse 15)?

One of the most famous examples of Solomon's wisdom is the story of two women who claimed to be the mother of the same baby. Read the details in 1 Kings 3:16-28. How did the way Solomon handled the situation reveal his wisdom?

How did the Israelites react to Solomon's decision (see verse 28)?

Now look at 1 Kings 4:29-34. How did people of other nations react to Solomon as a man of wisdom?

Solomon reigned many years and accomplished great things, including building a great Temple for God and a palace for himself. How many years did it take for Solomon to build God's Temple? How many years did it take him to build his own palace (see 1 Kings 6:38–7:1)?

It is possible that this is when Solomon started to get off track and make unwise decisions. Move on to 1 Kings 11:1-13. What did Solomon do that God had told the Israelites they must never do? To whom did Solomon begin to listen instead of God (see verses 2-4)?

What was God's reaction (see verses 9-13)?

Heavenly Father, I do not want to get focused on myself and forget You. Help me to always be guided by Your instructions and to stay on Your track of wisdom throughout my life. Amen.

Day 4: WISE COUNSEL VERSUS UNWISE COUNSEL

Lord, I need help when I am making decisions. Help me to live with my eyes on You, knowing that You will counsel me wisely as I seek You. Amen.

Decisions! What should I eat for lunch? Should I take this job or wait for a better offer? Should I stay in this relationship or break it off? We are constantly faced with decisions, big and small. Often when we are confronted by all of the decision-making we must do, we seek advice from trusted friends or self-help books. But we must learn how to seek wise counsel so that we can make decisions with understanding and discernment. The Bible reveals that we should seek God in our decision-making. Look at Jeremiah 29:11-13. What kinds of plans does God have for us (see verse 11)?

What does God promise to do when we call upon Him (see verse 12)?

What happens when we seek God with all our heart (see verse 13)?

Now turn to Psalm 16:7-8. How should we respond as we get wise counsel from the Lord?

The Bible reveals that we should also consult the special Counselor whom God sends to us. Read John 14:16-18. Who is this Counselor? How long will He be available to advise us?

Turn to Psalm 119:24,97-105. What else does God provide to counsel us?

What are some of the things that we gain from this counsel (see verses 98-101)?

Finally, the Bible reveals that we need to seek wise counsel from godly people in our lives. Read Proverbs 15:22. How does getting wise counsel from godly people affect our plans?

___

Lord, I want to seek Your counsel in everything I do. I will listen with open ears and an open heart to all the wise counsel that You provide for me. Amen.

Day 5 — ETERNAL VIEW VERSUS EARTHLY VIEW

Dear God, I want to know You and believe in You. Help me to understand who You are and how You love me. Draw me to surrender my heart and my life to You and You alone, focusing my view on eternity, not the world. Amen.

No matter how much we try in our own power to make wise decisions, we are sometimes going to mess up. As we apply ourselves to understanding how to make good decisions, we will obtain wisdom; but ultimately, we will fall short. We will still sometimes make wrong and unwise decisions. Fortunately, as believers we have made a decision that guides our eternal destinies—a decision that shapes our worldview and guides the way we live our lives each and every day. Read Romans 3:23. Why is it inevitable that we will all make some wrong decisions?

___

God does not leave us in this state of failure and discouragement. He knows that we are not perfect. He knows that we will sometimes fail to do the right thing, but He loves us anyway in spite of our failures. He loves us so much, in fact, that He made a way for us to have eternal life with Him, even though we don't deserve it. Read John 3:16-17. What did God do for us?

Why did God do this?

Read Romans 5:8. What exactly did Jesus do to save the world?

According to John 15:13, what did Jesus say about doing such a thing?

Do you grasp the magnitude of God's love for us? God's love for every one of us—me, you, every person—is so great that He sacrificed His Son for us. Jesus died to take the punishment that we deserve for our sins. According to Romans 10:9, what does someone have to do in order to be saved and have eternal life?

If all this is new for you, and if—after thinking about what has been presented here—you know that you want to declare your faith in Jesus and become a Christian, you must personally express your belief. Is this the desire of your heart right now? If so, pray the prayer below:

> *Dear God, I am ready to make the most important decision of my life. Forgive me for my unwise decisions of the past. Thank You for loving me so much that You would die for me so that I can have everlasting life. Take control of my life and make me the person You want me to be. Amen.*

You can be assured that Christ will come into your life just as He promised. Tell your Bible study leader that you prayed this prayer so that he or she can guide you to information that will help you grow in your new faith. If you are already a Christian, consider this day's study a reminder to you of God's redeeming love, and read Colossians 2:6-7. Because you have faith in Christ, what are you to do?

_____
_____
_____
_____

> *Dear God, thank You for Your great love and for the sacrifice of Your Son. Please forgive me when I make wrong decisions, and help me to have an eternal view of things, not an earthly view. Amen.*

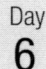
Day 6

REFLECTION AND APPLICATION

Dear Lord, I want to shine Your light out into this dark world today. Help me to be like Daniel and make wise decisions. Amen.

As you are out and about today, be intentional about shining God's light. Be proactive in talking to people and asking some questions that may lead to spiritual conversations—and get ready to shine as you hold out the word of truth! Here are some questions you can ask others to start the conversation:

1. What is the best decision you have ever made in your life?
2. Do you feel like you need wisdom beyond yourself when making big decisions?
3. What is your definition of wisdom?
4. Where do you look for wisdom?

If you listen—really listen—to what the other person says, you may discern that you can share what you believe about decision-making and godly wisdom. If God opens the door, take a step of faith and walk through it. Use the gospel presentation in Day 5 of this week's study if you get to a point in the conversation where you think the person is ready to hear how to accept Christ as his or her Savior.

Also, think about ways you can "shine" with wisdom without saying a word. How do you react when you're in a long line? Do you fret and fume, or do you practice a memory verse and patiently wait your turn? Do you always express a polite word of thanks when a friend or family member does something for you, or do you assume that because of your close relationship, you don't need to say anything? When you know someone is having a bad time, do you avoid the person, or do you try to think of something positive to say to or do for him or her? What are a few practical ways that you can quietly shine with wisdom in your part of the world?

_____

_____

_____

_____

Lord, prepare the hearts of those I meet to hear about godly wisdom that comes from You. Help me to use godly wisdom to shine Your light in many different ways. Amen.

Day 7

REFLECTION AND APPLICATION

God, I need to make fitness decisions today, and I need Your wisdom to guide me. Help me to put together an action plan based on wisdom from You. Amen.

Whether you have already established a fitness habit or you are just thinking about it, this is an area where wise decisions can positively impact your health. Consider the decision questions below, pray about each one as you reflect on its impact on your life, and then take the first step today to put these wise decisions into action. (Note: Remember to always consult a medical or health care professional before you begin any exercise or fitness routine.)

Decision Question #1: What types of exercise are you going to do? List all the various activities that come to mind, and then prioritize the listed items by what is the most appealing to you. Do not write down any type of fitness activity that you do not really want to do. Remember, you are deciding what you are *actually going* to do in your life.

_____
_____
_____

Decision Question #2: How often are you going to exercise during a week? Will it be every day, every other day, or just on weekdays? Write this down.

_____
_____
_____

Decision Question #3: What time of day will you exercise? Do you have the freedom to exercise early in the morning? What about during your lunch break? Or is evening the best time for you? Write down this time.

_____
_____
_____

Decision Question #4: How much time will you set aside to exercise? Will you start with 10 or 15 minutes, or jump right into a one-hour class? Do you want to exercise for several short periods of time during the day or exercise once for a longer period of time? Write down your plan.

_____

_____

_____

_____

Decision Question #5: What are you going to do to add a spiritual element to your fitness regime? Will you listen to a spiritual podcast? Worship music? What about using the time to practice your memory verses? Be creative and decide to have a time of spiritual reflection while you work on your physical fitness.

_____

_____

_____

_____

Now put together a plan of action based on these decisions, and start today! (If you need more help getting an exercise plan of action started, read the "Just Move" chapter in the *First Place 4 Health Member's Guide*.)

> *Heavenly Father, I know the power of wise decisions in the area of fitness. Help me to act on my decisions and put my plan into action. I want to build my strength in every area of my life so that I can be a shining light. Amen.*

Notes
1. Tassos Kioulachoglou, "The Fear of the Lord," *The Journal of Biblical Accuracy*. http://www.jba.gr/Articles/nkjv_jbaapr00a.htm (accessed January 2012).
2. *Merriam-Webster Online Dictionary*, www.merriam-webster.com, s.v. "understanding."

Group Prayer Requests

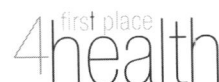

Today's Date: _____

Name	Request

Results

_____
_____
_____
_____
_____

Week Six

take small steps in the right direction

SCRIPTURE MEMORY VERSE
A prudent man gives thought to his steps.
PROVERBS 14:15

For better or worse, every little step we take adds to the one before it. All of our steps together—everything we do—make a difference somewhere.

In his book *The Slight Edge: Secret to a Successful Life*, author Jeff Olson shares this very philosophy that little steps compounded do make a difference. The things that we do every single day—even the things that don't look dramatic and don't appear to even matter—*do* matter. They not only make *a* difference, they make *all* the difference. Olson suggests that this philosophy will lead to simple actions, creating results that shape our lives.[1]

This week, we will look at various steps we take as we walk through life. Whether it is the first baby steps we take in a particular area of our lives or the running steps we take when we are in shape and moving fast, each step needs to be taken carefully and thoughtfully, knowing that God will keep us safe as long as we are walking and running in step with Him.

BAQY STEPS — Day 1

Lord, help me to be like a little child and take baby steps in the right direction. I know You will catch me when I fall, because You are my caring Father. Amen.

It's exciting when children take their first baby steps—for both the parents and the children. The parents are excited to see that their children are indeed growing, and the children are excited to be learning a new skill and to be "on their own," at least in a small sense. The children, of course, fall down, but they never hesitate to get back up and try again until they accomplish the mighty task of learning how to walk.

We adults, too, often need to "learn how to walk" in many areas of our lives. We need to take baby steps, for example, as we attempt to lead healthier lifestyles. Fortunately, God our Father is excited as we learn new skills. God wants us to succeed, and He will help us get back up and try again when we fall. He will be with us always. Read Romans 8:16. What are we in relation to God?

_____
_____
_____
_____

Turn to John 10:11-15. Just as a parent is a caretaker of his or her children, Jesus compared Himself to what other kind of caretaker?

_____
_____
_____
_____

Psalm 23 describes the path of life, with the Lord leading us. With what does the Lord provide us, and what happens to us as He leads us (see verses 1-2)?

_____
_____
_____

Along what path does God guide our steps (see verse 3)?

_____
_____
_____

Through what valley does God lead us step by step? Why should we be comforted as we take steps through it (see verse 4)?

_____
_____
_____

Where does God provide a table for us, and what is particularly significant about the location of this table?

_____
_____
_____

When we walk with God our Father, what will go along with us (see verse 6)?

_____
_____
_____

Ultimately, where will we dwell (see verse 6)?

_____
_____
_____

Loving Father, I need You to walk by my side as I take baby steps in many areas of my life. Pick me up when I fall. Lead me as a gentle shepherd. Amen.

STEADY SLOW STEPS

Day 2

Lord, help me to take time to be careful and wise in the steps I choose to take. Help me not to rush and take the wrong steps. Amen.

It takes patience to take slow steady steps when they are needed. Today, let's look at what we need to be disciplined to take those steady slow steps in the right direction. First, let's set the groundwork. Look at Proverbs 20:24. Who directs our steps?

That being true, why should we "give thought to" our steps (see our memory verse, Proverbs 14:15)?

The word "prudent" from this week's memory verse means "wise in handling practical matters; exercising good judgment or common sense."[2] What is the balance between prudently planning our steps and acknowledging that God is in control of our steps?

One character trait we need as we take steady slow steps is patience. We live in a society that wants results *now*. We want change *now*. And we want big changes, not small, simple-step changes. But there is value in patiently walking through life one step at a time with God determining the timeline. Read Psalm 40:1-3. What happens when we wait patiently for the Lord?

What does God do for us (see verses 2-3)?

What do God's actions accomplish aside from helping us (see verse 3)?

Read Galatians 5:22-25. Where is patience in this list (see verse 22)?

What is our connection to the Holy Spirit (see verse 25)?

When we "keep in step" with someone, we neither lag behind nor rush ahead. We walk side by side, step by step, together. How do we keep in step with the Holy Spirit?

Holy Spirit, I know that if I walk slowly and steadily by Your side, You will prompt me to grow the fruit of Your Spirit in me. Grant me Your strength as we walk together. Amen.

WEAK STEPS — Day 3

Heavenly Father, there are days when I don't even want to get out of bed, much less take any steps, no matter how small. Help me take the first step on days like this. Hold me up with Your strong arms. Amen.

What do we do on those days when it seems impossible to take even one step? What do we do when we don't seem to have the energy to even get out of bed, much less the strength to deal with what lies ahead? The answer is to remember what God says in His Word about where our strength comes from and on whom we can rely. Read 2 Corinthians 12:9-10. What are two things we are supposed to do concerning our weaknesses?

1. _____
2. _____

Why should we do these two things?
_____
_____
_____

According to Psalm 138:3, what should we do when we need strength?
_____
_____
_____

Read Ephesians 3:16. Who gives us strength? How do we receive His power?
_____
_____
_____

Read Romans 8:26-27. When we are so weak that we cannot even pray or don't know what to pray, who helps us? What does He do for us?
_____
_____
_____

Read Jeremiah 17:5. What did God say about relying "on flesh" for strength?
_____
_____
_____

What is the warning that Jeremiah gives?

We bless God by our willing spirit, even if our body is weak. God sends His Holy Spirit to be in us and give us strength and pray for us. He will walk with us through any valleys we face. Weak steps are better than no steps at all, so just take one step at a time. The Lord will be there with you.

Almighty Father, thank You for sending Your Holy Spirit to me. When I don't feel strong enough to move, I will take the first step, by faith, and trust that You will help me to take the next one. Amen.

STEEP STEPS — Day 4

Today, the road is steep and I need stamina to make it to the top, Lord. Help me to carefully prepare for the steep climb. I know You will be there with me as I climb. Amen.

Climbing walls is a popular sport. Maybe you've seen a climbing wall at such places as gyms, fairs or even birthday parties. Climbing is a different kind of workout and uses muscle groups unlike those used for everyday walking or running. In addition, just like anything else, when you do something you're not used to doing, you can end up pretty sore. Climbing is a challenge, both in fitness and in life. Because of this fact, you need to be both physically and *mentally* prepared for the climbs of life. Read 2 Corinthians 10:5. What action do we need to take regarding our thoughts?

How can we make our thoughts "obedient to Christ"?

What are a few specific ways you can align your thoughts with Christ?

What specifically gives you peace of mind as you climb? The answer is God, because He is your safety net. There is no better way to put it. Picture yourself hanging on the side of a cliff, held in place only by a rope and a few bolts and anchors. That's the way life is sometimes. We seem to be just barely hanging on. Now picture God at the bottom of the cliff, down below you. He is there as your safety net, and His arms are wide open. He simply asks that you follow His instructions in order to come down safely off the cliff. How is God described in Deuteronomy 33:26-27? Where specifically are His arms?

Read the following Scriptures and write down what it states about safety in each verse:

Scripture	What this says about safety
Lev. 25:18	
Job 5:11	
Ps. 12:7	

Scripture	What this says about safety
Ps. 37:3	
Prov. 1:33	
Prov. 28:26	

Now turn to Psalm 4. What should we *not* do when we are angry, frustrated or anxious about whatever climb we are facing (see verse 4)?

What *should* we do instead (see verse 5)?

What should give us confidence? Why should we feel this way (see verse 8)?

Mighty God, You are my safety net. You alone keep me safe when I climb the steep spots in life. I can always count on You to be there for me. Amen.

RUNNING STEPS — Day 5

God, grant me the energy to take running steps in my life. I feel the strength to move forward, yet I know this is not in my power but Yours. Amen.

As God strengthens us, we are readied for running steps in different areas of life. When He knows we are ready, He sets us free to feel the wind in our hair and the sweat on our bodies. It is hard work, this running; but this life is a race, and God wants us to run it with perseverance, trusting in Him. Look at Hebrews 12:1-3. Who are the people cheering us on in the race of life (see verse 1)?

What must we get rid of so that we can run more easily (see verse 1)?

Exactly how are we to run, and what does that mean?

Where should our focus be as we run, and why (see verse 2)?

How do we know that Jesus understands the perseverance we need (see verse 2)?

Considering what Jesus went through, how should we deal with any difficulties we face in life (see verse 3)?

Now read Isaiah 40:28-31. As we run the race of life, when is God available to help us? Why is this encouraging (see verse 28)?

How does God help us when we are weary (see verse 29)?

What does it take on our part (see verse 31)?

Dear Lord, I am so glad that I do not have to run this race of life on my own. Thank You for giving me strength. I will hold on to Your hand. Amen.

REFLECTION AND APPLICATION

Day 6

Lord, help me to take small action steps today and apply what I have been learning. Guide me and stay close to me as I step out in faith to do this. Amen.

All of us would love to be able to take quantum leaps in making changes in our lives, but the fact is that we must start with small steps. We can, however, have a "slight edge" as we start our race to improve our fitness in all areas of our lives. The following are some "slight edge" suggestions:

- Make it a point to actually use the memory verse cards that are provided at the back of this book. Take them with you as you exercise, do errands, drive your car. Practice the verses as you go. Write down on index cards other verses that you learn during this study that have particular personal meaning for you. Practice them along with the memory verses.

- Use a portable media player (such as an iPod) to listen to encouraging Christian music as you exercise. Sing or hum along and praise God each step of the way, no matter how long or short your fitness session is. (Of course, you don't have to wait to exercise to do this!)

- Wear a pedometer throughout the day and count how many "slight edge" steps you are taking beyond those you take when you exercise. You will be encouraged to see how the miles add up!

- Plan a "slight edge" celebration (such as visiting a park or museum or seeing a movie) once you have reached a set number of steps of walking, or establish some other short-term goal for yourself.

Be creative and think of other things you can do to have a slight edge as you take steps that will help you draw closer to God.

Thank You, Lord, for showing me how to take small steps in my race for life. Help me to be faithful to continue in this path of emotional, spiritual, mental and physical fitness every day. Amen.

REFLECTION AND APPLICATION

Day 7

Lord, You are a God who always keeps me safe. You also keep the loved ones in my life safe. You are the safety net that is always there, and I am grateful that I can always count on You. Thank You, Lord. Amen.

Think about how the concept of safety applies to every area of your life. What are some of the things that keep you emotionally safe?

_____
_____
_____

What are some of the things that keep you spiritually safe?

_____
_____
_____

What are some of the things that keep you mentally safe?

_____
_____
_____

What are some of the things that keep you physically safe?

_____
_____
_____

Heavenly Father, whether I am taking baby steps, steady slow steps, weak steps, steep steps or running steps, I know that You will always be with me. Guide my steps as I make every day my best day. Amen.

Notes

1. Jeff Olson, *The Slight Edge: Secret to a Successful Life* (Momentum Media, 2005).
2. *The American Heritage Dictionary of the English Language*, 2009 ed., s.v. "prudent," quoted at www.thefreedictionary.com (accessed February 2012).

Group Prayer Requests

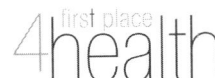

Today's Date: _____

Name	Request

Results

Week Seven

watch out for the father of lies

SCRIPTURE MEMORY VERSE
He has made everything beautiful in its time. He has also set eternity in the hearts of men; yet they cannot fathom what God has done from beginning to end.
ECCLESIASTES 3:11

This week we will focus on truth and lies. God, who "has made everything beautiful," is the light we live in, by and through. Satan, the father of lies, is a master of darkness and knows all the ways people can be deceived. In her book *The Lies Women Believe,* Nancy Leigh DeMoss points out that all of our problems started with a lie: "I want you to see how a lie was the starting place of all the trouble in the history of the universe. Eve listened to that lie, believed that lie, and acted on that lie."[1] She was deceived by the devil, and since that time, "Satan has used deception to win our affections, influence our choices, and destroy our lives."[2] God's plan, however, is for us to be freed by knowing the truth, because God has "set eternity" in our hearts. Let's get started pursuing truth and fleeing from lies!

DECEPTION VERSUS TRUTH

Day 1

Almighty God, I know You will guide me to truth and freedom. Help me to break free from any lies I have believed. I pray this in the name of Jesus. Amen.

The proper place to begin our study of lies is with the first lie ever told. Let's look at the story of Adam and Eve's encounter with Satan in the

Garden of Eden. Read Genesis 3:1-7. How is Satan, the devil who was disguised as a serpent, described (see verse 1)?

How did Satan begin to plant a seed of doubt in Eve's mind (see verse 1)?

What did Satan say that created doubt about God's goodness, love and motives (see verses 4-5)?

What was the result of this conversation (see verses 6-7)?

Sin began in the Garden of Eden with Satan's deception, but we can learn to recognize Satan's tricks, fight back against them and live in the truth—God's truth. Read John 8:44. What is the chief strategy of the devil?

Unfortunately, once we believe one of Satan's lies, we start on a downward spiral toward complete bondage, because believing the lie leads to dwelling on it, which in turn leads to acting on it. Read Romans 6:16. What is the difference between being enslaved to Satan through sin and being enslaved to God through obedience?

Read John 8:31-36. How are the disciples of Jesus to show that they are really His (see verse 31)?

To what does the truth lead (see verse 32)?

According to Jesus, how does someone break free from the bondage of sin (see verse 36)?

Dear God, I am ready to be set free. I want to live bonded to You through obedience. I will use Your truth to fight the deception that surrounds me. Amen.

Day 2 — OUTWARD BEAUTY VERSUS INNER BEAUTY

Lord, help me to see and believe the truth about Your love for me. I know that You see me as beautiful in this beautiful world You created. Amen.

Satan would have us believe that it is the world's ideas about beauty that should hold sway over our lives and everything we do—that our main goal should be to be beautiful on the outside. But this idea is just another attempt to deceive us. God's ideas about beauty are not the same as the world's (or Satan's) ideas. Read Ecclesiastes 3:11, the memory verse for this week. How many things has God made that are beautiful?

What has God set in people's hearts, and what exactly does that mean?

Ultimately, as great and beautiful as this world is, why is it unsatisfying for disciples of Jesus?

According to Proverbs 31:30, what happens to earthly beauty?

What sort of beauty is worthy of praise?

Read 1 Samuel 16:7. What about a person does God look at?

According to 1 Peter 3:3-4, from where should our beauty come?

Read Isaiah 52:7 and Romans 10:15. What is described as beautiful in these verses? Why are they beautiful?

According to Ephesians 6:15, with what are our feet to be fitted?

Father in heaven, I want the lasting beauty of eternity with You. Help me to ignore the lies about beauty that Satan and the world tell me. Guide me to know well what You have in my heart. Amen.

Day 3 — SINNING VERSUS RESISTING

Father, I know that Satan comes after me like a roaring lion. Help me to stand firm against his noisy assaults. I know that in You I can have victory. Amen.

We have an active part to play when it comes to opposing the strategies of Satan. Read 1 Peter 5:8-9. What does the devil spend his time doing?

In what ways does Satan try to "devour" us?

According to verse 9, how should we resist Satan?

Read Ephesians 4:25-27. What things should we avoid (see verses 25-26)?

What happens when we disobey God (see verse 27)?

Read Luke 4:1-13. How did Jesus resist the devil when Satan tempted Him in the wilderness (see verses 4,8,12)?

_____
_____
_____

We, too, are tempted, but there is hope for resisting the temptation if we are alert to it. Read 1 Corinthians 10:13. In what two ways does God help us whenever we are tempted to give in to sin?

1. _____
2. _____

According to James 4:7, what will happen when we resist the devil and his temptations?

_____
_____
_____

Lord, help me to resist the devil so that he will flee from me. I know You will not allow me to be tempted beyond what I can handle. Amen.

PRAYER VERSUS TEMPTATION

Day 4

Mighty God, I know that You hear my prayers, and I know that prayer is a key part of overcoming the enemy's tactics in my life. Help me to be faithful to always turn to prayer when I am under attack. Amen.

There is power in prayer—power that can help you defeat the enemy, the devil, when he comes roaring after you. Read Matthew 26:41. What is the warning here?

_____
_____
_____

In Ephesians 6:10-17, Paul lists some of the spiritual armor we need to wear when we battle the enemy. There is one more item that is necessary in our battle, though it is not a particular piece of armor: prayer. Read Ephesians 6:18. How often are we supposed to pray?

For whom are we supposed to pray?

David had a close relationship to God and often talked to Him in prayer. Read Psalm 86, one of the fervent prayers David said when he was in need. What did David ask for in each of the following verses, and why did David expect God to answer each of his requests positively?

Scripture	David's request	What David did
Ps. 86:2		
Ps. 86:3		
Ps. 86:4		

According to verses 5-7, why does God answer prayer?

_____
_____
_____

Why is our God the one true God (see verses 8-10)?

_____
_____
_____

What did David want God to do after He answered his prayer? What did David say he would do (see verses 11-13)?

_____
_____
_____
_____

Lord, I want to draw close to You in prayer and talk to You like the caring father that You are. Help me to share honest prayers with You like David did, asking for Your help and sharing that I am trying to do my part. Amen.

LIGHT VERSUS DARKNESS

Day 5

Dear God, You are the light of the world. I want to walk in the light of Your love so that I, too, can shine Your light in the darkness. Amen.

Satan always wanted to be like God. In Isaiah 14:13, we read that Satan said, "I will ascend to heaven; I will raise my throne above the stars of God; I will sit enthroned on the mount of assembly, on the utmost heights of the sacred mountain." He wanted to be light like God, but he is darkness, and we need to be careful and not be taken in by his deceptive ways. Read 1 John 1:5-7. What is God's relationship to light (see verse 5)?

What is true for us if we continue to walk in darkness (see verse 6)?

What is true for us if we walk in the light (see verse 7)?

Read 2 Corinthians 11:14-15. As what do Satan and his servants masquerade? What impact does this have on those who wish to walk in God's true light?

According to 1 Peter 2:9, who called us out of the darkness?

Read Matthew 5:14-16. What did Jesus call His disciples, and what did He tell them to do?

When we do what Jesus said to do, what will happen (see verse 16)?

Dear Lord, I want to shine Your light and give You glory each and every day. Help me to be alert to the opportunities that come my way so that I don't miss any opportunity to show others who You are. Amen.

REFLECTION AND APPLICATION

Day 6

Dear God, I am thankful that I am Yours and that You love me and have set eternity in my heart. Help me as I seek to know You better and make every day my best day. Amen.

One of the points of our memory verse is that God's actions, thoughts, emotions—everything about God—are actually beyond our capacity to understand. We simply cannot comprehend all that God is, has done and plans to do. Read what Job 11:7-9 has to say:

> Can you fathom the mysteries of God? Can you probe the limits of the Almighty? They are higher than the heavens—what can you do? They are deeper than the depths of the grave—what can you know? Their measure is longer than the earth and wider than the sea.

God's knowledge is so vast and limitless that no one on earth could ever match it. Paul said something similar about God's love:

> I pray that you, being rooted and established in love, may have power, together with all the saints, to grasp how wide and long and high and deep is the love of Christ, and to know this love that surpasses knowledge—that you may be filled to the measure of all the fullness of God (Ephesians 3:17-19).

We know what God's love is because we've seen it in action: He sacrificed His only Son for us. But God's love is so immense that we cannot really know everything about it. God's love is immeasurable, as is His wisdom:

> Where then does wisdom come from? Where does understanding dwell? It is hidden from the eyes of every living thing, concealed even from the birds of the air. Destruction and Death say, "Only a rumor of it has reached our ears." God understands the way to it and he alone knows where it dwells, for he views the ends of the earth and sees everything under the heavens. When he established the force of the wind and measured out the waters, when he made a decree for the rain and a path for the thunderstorm, then he looked at wisdom and appraised it; he confirmed it and tested it (Job 28:20-27).

All knowledge, love and wisdom have been with God from the very beginning. And the really incredible thing—what *really* is beyond belief—is that God wants to share it all with us!

Take several minutes today to think about the immeasurable knowledge and wisdom God has and thank Him for making a lot of it available in the Bible, His Word. Also try to imagine the size and scope of God's love for you. Yes, He loves everyone, but take a few minutes and really try to imagine the love God has for you alone. Sit quietly and let God's love quiet any worries you have. Let it encourage you and protect you from evil. Let it lift you up so that you make this day and every day your best day.

Lord, all of Your ways may be beyond my understanding, but I want to try to know You better and better, to the best of my ability. I look forward to the day I will see and know You in heaven. Amen.

REFLECTION AND APPLICATION

Day 7

Lord, help me to speak words of encouragement to those who need to know they are loved by You. Bring people across my path who need to know You and Your amazing grace. Amen.

This week's memory verse tells a simple truth: God makes everything beautiful in its time, and we are all beautiful in God's eyes. All people need to know this. We can help to spread the word by shining God's light in a world darkened by Satan's lies and deceptions. We can share with others the eternity that God has set in our hearts. We can play a positive role in bringing God's truth to all of the people—family, friends, even strangers—in whatever part of the world we live, no matter how large or small our niche is in the world.

As you go through your day today, see how many people you can encourage in an honest, loving way. It might be a comment you make to a complete stranger or something you say to someone in your family. It might be a compliment to a senior citizen or to a little child or a parent. You might open the door for someone or let someone ahead of you in line. At the very least, try smiling at everyone you meet. You never know when even a smile may brighten someone's day and encourage that person.

The point is that you should show God's love to everyone that crosses your path. An encouraging word or an act of kindness shows God's love to the world. At the very least, your words or actions may cause someone else to want to learn more about why you can speak and act the way you do, leading to your being able to have a conversation about God's love and His kingdom!

What are some ways you can encourage some of your family members?

What are some ways you can encourage some of your friends?

What are some ways you can encourage other members of your First Place 4 Health group?

What are some ways you can encourage strangers whom you might meet during the day?

Who are others in your life who need a word of encouragement today? How will you continue to share the light of God with those you meet?

_____
_____
_____
_____

Heavenly Father, thank You for opportunities to encourage others by showing them Your love. Help me to guide them to take one step closer to You as I shine Your light out to them through my words and actions. Amen.

Notes
1. Nancy Leigh DeMoss, *Lies Women Believe: And the Truth That Sets Them Free* (Chicago: Moody Publishers, 2002), p. 20.
2. Ibid., p. 32.

Group Prayer Requests

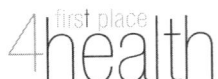

Today's Date: _____

Name	Request

Results

_____
_____
_____
_____
_____

Week Eight

get your spiritual life in shape

SCRIPTURE MEMORY VERSE

I will sing of the LORD's great love forever; with my mouth I will make your faithfulness known through all generations. I will declare that your love stands firm forever, that you established your faithfulness in heaven itself.

PSALM 89:1-2

Getting our spiritual lives in shape requires a conscious effort on our part. It's all too easy to get caught up in doing things and going places. We start out great, anxious to take part in church committees and missions, join the choir, and go to every Bible study we can find. But then the things of the world distract us. Our enthusiasm fades, and we begin to think that going to church on Sunday is enough (as long as there's no important game on TV, or our kids don't have soccer, or there isn't some other essential thing going on we can't miss). We begin to slide by, thinking that God will understand. After all, we still have faith in Jesus, right? *Right?*

God wants more time with us than just on Sunday. He wants us to continue to grow and act out our faith so that we will serve as a light for Him in this world. To do that, we need to get our spiritual lives in shape by prioritizing our time with God, our time studying His Word and our time with His people. It is tempting to get busy with other things in life and neglect our spiritual fitness. But we need to focus on God and remember His love and His faithfulness—a love and faithfulness that we should return. Then we will praise God and stay focused so that we can grow spiritually.

Day 1

DRAW NEAR TO GOD

Lord, I know that I will grow spiritually if I stay close to You. I want to learn to cling to You during the good times and the bad times. Draw me near to You, O God. Thank You, Heavenly Father. Amen.

The busyness of day-to-day life can distract us from the priorities that God has set for us. But making every day our best day necessarily means making God an integral part of everything we do. We do that by drawing near to Him on a daily basis. Read Hebrews 10:19-23. What does this passage call us to do (see verse 22)?

_____
_____
_____
_____

Why can we have confidence to do this (see verses 19-21)?

_____
_____
_____
_____

What are the four conditions we need to meet in order to do this (see verse 22)?

1. _____
2. _____
3. _____
4. _____

To what are we to hold on, and what exactly is this (see verse 23)?

_____
_____
_____

Why can we have this (see verse 23)?

_____
_____

What are two practical ways to "hold unswervingly to the hope"?

1. _____
2. _____

Read Psalm 32:7 and James 4:8. When we draw near to God, what will He do for us?

_____
_____
_____

Lord, I want Your presence to be a part of my daily life. Help me to not be swayed by the busyness of life so that I neglect You and Your teachings. Amen.

GROW BY PRAYING — Day 2

Lord, help me to create a daily habit of praying. You are an awesome God who can hear all of us praying at the same time. What a chorus that must be!

We know that prayer is a discipline of the Christian life. We know that there is power in prayer. We know that to connect to God, we need to pray. We also know that when we pray, we need to be focused on God. We "know" so much, yet we often fail to do what will grow our faith and bring us closer to God. We *need* to pray—constantly, faithfully and expectantly. Look up 1 Thessalonians 5:16-18. What three things are we urged to do?

1. _____
2. _____
3. _____

Why are we to do these things (see verse 18)?

Why can Christians always be joyful—regardless of our circumstances?

What advantages are there in praying regularly?

According to James 4:10, what will God do for us when we pray?

What did Jesus say God would do when we pray (see Matthew 6:6)?

Read John 15:5. Why should we stay connected to God?

If we want to grow more connected to God—if we want to get to know Him better—we must pray to Him. It's as simple as that.

Dear heavenly Father, it blesses me to know that You hear my prayers. Help me to grow in my prayer life so that I can be a person who prays continually, confident You will answer. Amen.

READ GOD'S WORD DAILY

Day 3

Lord, I know I need to read Your holy Word every day. I understand that it is Your love letter to me and I should treasure it. Help me to be faithful in making the study of Your Word a priority. Thank You, Lord. Amen.

Do you start the day with God's Word? Do you read it off and on throughout the day? Do you read it with your family? Do you read it as the last thing you do before going to bed? Any (or all) of these is a great option. The important thing is to *read* it every day. If we don't make it part of our daily spiritual discipline, it will slip away from us, and we will lose sight of what we should be doing and why we should be doing it. We will lose a connection to God.

Joining a Bible study like the one of which you're currently a member is a great way to create accountability in the area of Bible reading. In order to receive the benefits of the study, however, you need to stay up to date with the reading. It is a good thing! One of the most powerful passages of Scripture concerning God's Word is Psalm 119. You read some of this psalm back in Week Five, but now read all of it. How do we know the right way to live (see verse 9)?

_____

_____

_____

What should we commit to do (see verses 10,17)?

_____

_____

_____

What helps us avoid sin, and how do we do this (see verses 11,13)?

How should we feel about following God's instructions (see verses 14-16)?

What does the psalmist ask of God (see verse 18)?

Besides giving us God's instructions, what does the Bible tell us about His Word (see verses 49-50,65)?

How do we learn to understand God's Word (see verse 73)?

What are three things that we gain from reading God's Word (see verses 98-100)?

1.
2.
3.

In light of what you learned in Week Seven about Satan, the father of lies, what else does God's Word help us to do (see verse 105)?

_____
_____
_____
_____
_____

Memorizing Scripture—hiding God's Word in our hearts—is an important spiritual discipline that is part of the First Place 4 Health program. For each week, commit to being faithful to practice the memory verse every day so that it will find a place in your heart and be available anytime you need it.

> *Heavenly Father, thank You for the light of Your Word that shines in my life. Help me to hide it in my heart so that I will not sin against You and so that I will find hope in Your promises. Amen.*

LIFT YOUR HEART IN WORSHIP — Day 4

> *Lord, I love to sing praises to You. I know it blesses You, and it blesses me as well. I worship You because You are worthy of my praise! Amen.*

When we think of worship, the first thing that often comes to mind is music. For centuries people have been pouring out their hearts to God in a variety of different forms of music styles, and today there is a large amount of contemporary Christian music available on the market. The variety of worship music is so vast, in fact, that almost everyone can find some type that he or she enjoys.

Music, however, is just one form of worship. There are probably as many different forms of worship as there are styles of music, and the Bible mentions many of them. Read the following verses on the next page and write down what way of worship is suggested.

Scripture	Type of worship
Ps. 34:1	
Ps. 47:1	(1)
	(2)
Ps. 63:4	
Ps. 95:1	(1)
	(2)
Ps. 95:2	
Ps. 95:6	(1)
	(2)
Ps. 119:120	
Ps. 149:3	(1)
	(2)

Reread this week's memory verse, Psalm 89:1-2. What ways to worship God are mentioned?

_____
_____
_____
_____

Read Hebrews 12:28-29. Although there are many ways to worship God, what did the writer of Hebrews say about how we should worship?

_____
_____
_____
_____

Turn to John 4:21-24. During Jesus' time, the Samaritans' version of the Bible had only the first five books of the Bible, so unlike the Jews, they knew little if anything about the Messiah who was to come. The Samaritans also differed with the Jews about where the proper place was to worship God. According to Jesus, when will all people worship God the same way (see verse 21)?

Why won't the place of worship matter?

What kind of worshipers does God seek, and why (see verses 23-24)?

Dear God, I want to worship You in spirit and in truth. I want to worship You in all of the splendor of Your majesty. Help me, Lord, to be faithful to bring true worship to You every day. Thank You, Lord. Amen.

MEET IN FELLOWSHIP

Day 5

Heavenly Father, I want to spend time with others who believe in You. Help me to be an encouragement to them as they in turn encourage me. Amen.

It is so great to spend time with others who have the same worldview as we do. When we meet with fellow believers, we feel as if we are with family—and that is exactly as we should feel, for we are all sons and daughters in the family of God. Read Ecclesiastes 4:9-12. What are two important reasons that fellowship is good for us?

___

Turn to Acts 4:34-37. How was fellowship practiced in the Early Church?

___

Read 1 Corinthians 12:12-27. What is it that binds together all believers (see verse 13)?

___

What does a person's body need to function properly (see verses 14-20)?

___

Why should we have fellowship with other believers (see verses 24-27)?

___

Read Hebrews 10:24-25. What are the three things that the writer of Hebrews says the members of the Body of Christ should do?

1. ___
2. ___
3. ___

According to John 17:20-21, what did Jesus pray for His disciples, and what is one very important thing that this would accomplish?

_____

_____

Lord, thank You for the fellowship we have with You and with each other. Continue to teach me that I can be stronger when I have fellowship with other members of the Body and that we can function better together. Amen.

REFLECTION AND APPLICATION

Day 6

Dear Lord, I know the power of Your Word and the importance of hiding it in my heart. Help me to be faithful to memorize Your Word. I want to learn from Your Word and use it in my life. Amen.

One of the things on which we focused during this week was the importance of studying God's Word and memorizing verses from it. So now is an appropriate time to review all of our memory verses we have covered so far. Write out each verse from memory, and then note at least one new thing you have learned from it.

Memory verse	What I have learned
Isaiah 43:18:	
Matthew 6:34:	
Psalm 31:14-15:	

Memory verse	What I have learned
Psalm 111:10:	
Proverbs 14:15:	
Ecclesiastes 3:11:	
Psalm 89:1-2:	

If at any time you doubt the effectiveness of memorizing Scripture, remind yourself of how Jesus dealt successfully with Satan during the temptation in the wilderness (see Matthew 4:1-11; Luke 4:1-13).

Thank You, Lord, for giving us Your Word to guide us. Help me to hide it in my heart so that I will not sin against You, so that I can resist the enemy's attacks, and so I am always reminded of Your love and Your promises. Amen.

Day 7 — REFLECTION AND APPLICATION

Lord, help me to develop a worshipful attitude in all that I do. I want to thank You throughout the day for the things You do for me, and I want to share You with others, encouraging them to seek You and worship You. Amen.

Worship touches the heart of God, and making worship something you do every day is of prime importance in your Christian walk. Worship not only glorifies God for all of His mighty works, but it will also lift your heart and mind above the hardships, troubles and problems of this world.

If you have not already done so, begin today to make worship a daily habit—not just something you do in church on Sundays or just in the morning on the other days of the week. Listen to a Christian radio station when you are in the car, walk with an iPod playing your favorite worship songs, or play a CD of Christian worship songs on your home music system. Sing as you listen to the music, or hum along. Praise God during the day as you find things for which to be thankful. And try worshiping God in a manner different from your usual ways. If you're used to kneeling in worship, try standing and lifting your hands. If you're used to standing, try bowing low to the ground, or lay facedown on the floor.

Figure out ways to make worship something you can't live without on a day-to-day basis. On some days, it just may be the best part of your day!

What are a few specific ways that you will incorporate worship in your day-to-day activities?

_____
_____
_____
_____
_____

What is one new manner in which you will worship?

_____
_____
_____
_____
_____

Heavenly Father, thank You for showing me the importance of worship and the many ways I can worship You. Help me to be faithful to grow daily by praising You for all of Your gifts to me. I am so very thankful for Your love. Amen.

Group Prayer Requests

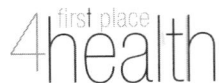

Today's Date: _____

Name	Request

Results

Week Nine

take care of your physical health

SCRIPTURE MEMORY VERSE
Train yourself to be godly. For physical training is of some value, but godliness has value for all things, holding promise for both the present life and the life to come.
1 TIMOTHY 4:7-8

Sometimes we might wonder why God placed us here in these fragile human bodies. We can easily injure ourselves—we can cut ourselves on the edge of a piece of paper, to say nothing about what happens if we fall down a flight of stairs. We can get sick—we may have to contend with anything from a simple cold to a major illness like cancer. We can have emotional problems—we can be hurt by anything as simple as one unkind word or suffer emotional turmoil when we have to deal with a broken relationship or what seems like overwhelming grief when a loved one dies.

Yes, we probably will experience many problems because of these earthly bodies, but God knew what He was doing when He created us. We just need to learn how best to take care of what God has given to us. This week, we will look at various aspects of how to take care of our bodies, searching the Scriptures for why we need to be concerned that our hearts are healthy, that we get our strength and flexibility from the proper sources, and that we provide ourselves with good nutrition and peaceful sleep. Even though godliness has more lasting value than physical training, God wants us to care as much as He does about our fitness in all areas of our lives. That's part of how we make every day our best day!

Day 1

GUARD YOUR HEART

Lord, help me to gain perspective this week on how and why I am supposed to take care of my body. Help me to trust You as I do my best to seek personal health in all areas of my life. Amen.

Before we focus on our hearts, we need to take an overall look at the relationship between physical health and spiritual wellbeing. We need to gain the right perspective and see the contrast between the two. Read 1 Timothy 4:7-8, the memory verse for this week. Although both physical training and godly training are necessary, which is more important, and why?

According to Titus 1:1, what leads to godliness?

Turn to 1 Timothy 3:16. What (or who) is the truth, the "mystery of godliness"?

How do we reveal whether we know the truth (see Matthew 12:34-35)?

Read Proverbs 4:23. Why is it so important that we guard our hearts?

According to Proverbs 27:19, what does the heart "reflect"?

Read Mark 7:20-23. What will our hearts reveal if we have not guarded them?

What we have in our hearts reveals what we have stored there, and what we have stored there affects our spiritual health. According to Proverbs 17:22, how does what we have stored in our hearts affect us physically?

What are a few practical ways to guard our hearts?

Lord, I want to have a strong heart physically, spiritually, mentally and emotionally. Help me to work these areas with a "cheerful heart" attitude.

Day 2

GAIN STRENGTH

Heavenly Father, I want to be strong in Your mighty power. I know that I cannot do anything through my own power. I want to be able to carry out Your work here on earth and wisely share Your love with others. Amen.

Have you ever been on a mission trip that included a building project? If you have, you know it takes physical strength to serve the Lord in such situations. If you are serving the Lord by caring for your family, you realize that you need strong arms to carry children, groceries and laundry and/or the physical stamina to go off to the workplace every day and deal with whatever occurs. God wants us to be strong in many ways. Read Joshua 1:6-9. Why could Joshua be strong (see verse 9)?

What condition did God give Joshua for his success (see verses 7-8)?

Read Ephesians 6:10-12. Who gives us power to be strong (see verse 10)?

Why is this sort of power necessary (see verse 12)?

Read Ephesians 1:18-20, part of Paul's prayer for the Ephesians. Because of His incredible power, what was God able to do (see verse 20)?

_____
_____
_____

Where is God's incredible power at work now (see verse 19)?

_____
_____
_____

Read Philippians 4:13. Whenever we feel weak—in any area of our lives—why should we be encouraged to go on?

_____
_____
_____

When we face any sort of battle, in whose strength should we operate, and where can we turn to learn how we should wage the fight?

_____
_____
_____

Lord, help me to be strong and stand firm. I need Your strength for all the battles I face. Thank You for always being there for me. Amen.

BE FLEXIBLE — Day 3

Lord, I know You want to stretch me in my faith. I know that this will require me to be flexible in many ways. Help me to follow Your lead as I strive to grow in this area. Amen.

One of the forms of exercise that is often neglected is flexibility training. Why is that? Maybe it is because we don't see immediate results. We don't see the sweat like we experience when we go through a cardio workout. We don't feel the burn like we do when we practice strength training. As we push our stretching and flexibility limits, sometimes all we experience is muscle soreness. What fun is that?

The basic principle of flexibility training is that stretching a muscle creates micro-tears that allow for the desired stretching to occur. Life is like this as well. Micro-tears need to happen for us to grow and have a more flexible life that trusts in God's guidance. Being flexible means letting go of control and allowing God to be in charge. There is a peace that comes with this that passes understanding. It is worth the pain. Read Genesis 12:1-5. What did Abram do, and why did he do it?

_____
_____
_____

Read Matthew 2:7-12. What did the Magi do to show that they were flexible, and why did they do it (see verse 12)?

_____
_____
_____

According to Mark 1:16-20, what did Simon, Andrew, James and John do to show that they were flexible?

_____
_____
_____

Read 1 Samuel 15:1-29. What happened when King Saul was stubborn and did things his own way, instead of how God had instructed him?

_____
_____
_____

Read Luke 10:38-41. How was the flexibility of Mary different from that of Martha?

According to David, whose will should we be doing (see Psalm 40:8)?

Read 2 Corinthians 4:7-18. Why was it appropriate that Paul compare us to clay jars (see verse 7)?

How did Paul say the believers were being "stretched" (see verses 8-9,16)?

Ultimately, what is the goal of all of this stretching and flexibility training (see verses 14,17)?

Dear God, I want to be flexible and let You show me how I should live my life. Stretch me so that I can see where I need more training. Encourage me as I become more adaptable to Your control. Amen.

Day 4

FUEL YOUR BODY

Lord, guide me to recognize that I need food to fuel my body, not to give me comfort. My real comfort comes from You. Help me to understand that the only thing that matters is You. Thank You for guiding my life. Amen.

Food is not supposed to be our source of happiness. It is not meant to be what comforts us. It is fuel—fuel to keep us growing and going forward for the Lord's purposes. God is our joy and our comfort. We need to embrace this truth and get a new perspective on eating. Read 1 Corinthians 10:31–11:1. As we fuel our bodies, what purpose should we have in mind?

_____

What should be the aim of everything that we do (see verse 33)?

_____

Why should we follow Paul's example (see verse 11:1)?

_____

Read 1 Corinthians 8:4-13, which is part of Paul's discussion about eating food that had been sacrificed to idols. Why did Paul say that the believers in Corinth could eat such food (see verse 4)?

_____

What did Paul say about the relationship between food and God (see verse 8)?

Why, though, could eating such food be a problem (see verses 7, 9-13)?

According to Isaiah 55:2 and Hebrews 6:5, on what should we really feast?

Although it is our souls that we should seek most to nourish, why should how we nourish our bodies also be important (see 1 Corinthians 6:19-20)?

Lord, help me to gain Your perspective on how I should nourish myself.
I want my body to be a healthy and holy place for Your dwelling.
Help me to make wise eating choices every day, to Your glory! Amen.

Day 5

GET SOME REST

Heavenly Father, I know I need times of rest with You in order to be at my best to serve You. Help me to figure out how to prioritize this in my busy life.

Rest. The mere word evokes longing in most of our hearts! The majority of us live busy lives, and there hardly seems to be enough time to do all the things we need to do, much less get enough rest. But even God rested on the seventh day of creation, so He modeled for us that we need to step back from our busyness and take the time to rest. Read Exodus 20:8-11 and Deuteronomy 5:12-15. Who is to honor the Sabbath, and how exactly are we to treat it as holy?

Read Mark 6:30-31. Why did Jesus suggest that He and His followers needed to rest?

Turn to Matthew 11:28-29. Where did Jesus say we should go for rest, and why?

What did Jesus suggest that we should do in order to rest (see verse 29)?

According to Psalm 62:1, where did David find rest?

According to Jeremiah 6:16, how will we find rest?

Read Matthew 8:23-27. What was troubling the disciples (see verses 24-25)?

What did Jesus do for His disciples, and what will He do when we need to rest from the storms of life (see verse 26)?

Dear Lord, thank You for setting the example of prioritizing rest. Help me to examine my life and make time for rest as well. I know rest will make me stronger and healthier in all areas of my life. Amen.

REFLECTION AND APPLICATION

Day 6

Dear Lord, help me to focus on the most important message You have for me from this week's study. Speak to me from Your Word and guide my steps to physical and spiritual health. Amen.

The human heart is indispensible for our earthly life. If we are going to live with vitality, serving God and sharing His message of truth in a fallen world, we need to have strong hearts. The healthy state of our heart reflects the discipline we have in the area of physical training, and the discipline we have in this area bubbles over to discipline in other areas of our lives. If we lack fitness in any area, it's hard to shine our light for the Lord.

Take a few minutes to consider the present condition of your heart. For each area of your life, briefly describe what you are currently doing to guard and strengthen your heart. Then list at least one specific thing that you can start to put into practice to improve your fitness in each area.

	What I'm doing	What I can put into practice
Emotionally		
Spiritually		
Physically		
Mentally		

Thank You, God, for helping me know how to guard and strengthen my heart. It blesses me to know that You care for me in that personal way. I know that my fitness in every area of my life will grow as You continue to guide me. I look to You for help! Amen.

REFLECTION AND APPLICATION

Day 7

Lord, I need You to guide me one step at a time to take action to make time for rest. Help me to communicate this need to my family and to help them seek and find times of rest as well. Amen.

Aside from observing Sunday as a day of rest, we all need to find times and places to rest with God on a daily basis. Although finding times to rest may prove to be elusive and will probably vary according to our season in life, we still must find time to rest with God every day. It is God who is our strength, and without God, we can do nothing. Before trying to examine how to add times for rest in your life, you need to answer some personal questions. Start with the questions listed here and then add any you think of that are relevant for you.

Are you single or married? Are you a caregiver? Do you have responsibilities to fulfill for others?

_____
_____
_____

Do you work part time or full time? How does this affect your schedule?

_____
_____
_____

What is your commute like? How much time does that take up?

_____
_____
_____

What are your commitments at church? Are you finding joy in serving? Why or why not?

What other obligations do you have to fulfill (volunteer work, school attendance, and the like)?

After taking a look at the reality of where you are in life, now consider how you can make sure that you have quiet time alone with God. When is the best time for you to have a spiritual rest, to pray and to read and study the Bible? Can you plan a longer time slot on days when you have fewer responsibilities to fulfill?

Where can you set up a place of spiritual rest in your home—a place (preferably with a door you can close) where you keep your Bible and study materials, your journal and whatever else you need for your time alone with God?

When do you have time for physical rest (taking a nap, having a massage, sitting in a room by yourself)? How often is it reasonable to expect to do this?

_____
_____
_____
_____

When can you make time for emotional rest (such as a getaway with your spouse or one or two friends)? How can you go about planning this sort of rest?

_____
_____
_____
_____

When can you take time for a mental rest where you don't have to think about work or any other responsibility? What do you enjoy doing that makes your mind rest and your worries quiet (read a book, do a puzzle, listen to music)?

_____
_____
_____
_____

If you think you can't find the time to take the rest that you need, remember it was God who set our example to follow. If God could take the time to rest (and He did!), so can you. Recall what this week's memory verse says: "Train yourself to be godly.... Godliness has value for all things."

God, You have set Yourself as an example for me to follow in all things, so I will take the time to rest—in every area of life. I want to honor You and glorify You and be blessed by You. Help me make every day my best day. Amen.

Group Prayer Requests

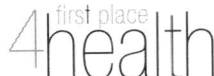

Today's Date: _____

Name	Request

Results

Week Ten

guard your heart and emotions daily

SCRIPTURE MEMORY VERSE
We have this hope as an anchor for the soul, firm and secure.
HEBREWS 6:19

Have you ever been in a position where you could tell that what was being said or how people were reacting could cause damage to your heart emotionally? Have you ever heard about a problem that someone was having and responded by saying, "That is heartbreaking"? When our emotions are touched by difficult circumstances, we may feel as if our hearts are breaking. And when the turmoil or difficulty is particularly painful emotionally, we sometimes have a physical reaction as well.

This week, we are going to spend time examining how David reached up to God. David was an emotional guy, and he knew how to pour his heart out before his God and express his emotions honestly—emotions to which we all can relate. He had such a close relationship to God that he even felt comfortable asking the Lord questions. And he certainly recognized where all of his good gifts came from, so he openly and regularly praised and thanked God. David is a great example for us to follow.

DEAL WITH DESPAIR

Day 1

Lord, help me to find hope in my brokenhearted moments. Help me to shine Your hope into the lives of others who are also brokenhearted. Amen.

God is near to all of us all of the time. We perhaps especially feel this close connection when we are overcome by despair or grief. When we feel brokenhearted, it is God who brings us hope. He expects us to depend on Him, because we *can*. Read Psalm 34:17-18. To whom is God close, and what does He do for them?

_____
_____
_____
_____

Look up Psalm 51:16-17. What does God love more than sacrifices? Why?

_____
_____
_____
_____

Although not written by David, Psalm 147:3 also tells us what God does for the brokenhearted. What is it that God does?

_____
_____
_____
_____

Read 2 Samuel 22:5-7. How did David feel when his enemies were all around him?

_____
_____
_____

Now read Psalm 18:16-24. What did God do for David when David felt despair (see verses 16-20)?

_____
_____
_____
_____

Why was God pleased with David (see verses 19-24)?

Hope is one of the critical emotions that will help us to rise above the tragedies and troubles of life. In Hebrews 6:19, the memory verse for this week, the writer provides us with a great message of hope. What is the picture of hope in this verse?

What does an anchor do for a boat? Why does hope act as an anchor?

Who guarantees our safety, no matter what happens to us or how badly others hurt us? How?

Let's determine to be a people who live out the hope we have and share it with others!

> *Lord, I want to be a person of hope! I want to help heal the brokenhearted. Heal my hurts and lead me through my times of despair so that I can better serve others. Than You, Lord. Amen.*

Day 2 — BE HONEST WITH GOD

Lord, help me to continually be honest with You about all of my emotions. I lay them at Your feet and trust them to You with all my heart. Amen.

David is one of the most honest people in the Bible. He was not perfect by any means, but he was not afraid to pour out to God exactly how he felt. He was honest with God, and we also can be honest with God about how we feel. Yesterday, you read part of Psalm 18. Now read all of it. Today we will look at each section of this psalm, which David wrote when the Lord delivered him from his enemies and from Saul, the king of Israel. How did David begin this psalm (see verses 1-3)?

In what sort of situation did David find himself (see verses 4-5)?

When David was distressed, what did he do, and what happened (see verse 6)?

What does David describe in verses 7-15?

As we discussed yesterday, in Psalm 18:16-24, David described how and why God had helped him. What message does David share in verses 25-29?

How does David describe God in verses 30-36?

According to verses 37-45, how did David's situation play out?

How did David end this psalm (see verses 46-50)?

Pretty powerful stuff, yes? During this intense emotional time, God was there for David, and David was not afraid to be honest and express his emotions in a song that would be sung before many. Even though the battles David engaged in were fierce, David knew God was on his side. He never doubted that God was able to rescue him, and God proved Himself faithful. We can be as honest with God as David was, and God will be just as faithful with us.

Lord, whether I am happy or sad, laughing or grieving, I can share what I feel with You. I can trust You to be with me and rescue me in every situation.

Day 3

MAKE REQUESTS OF GOD

Lord, thank You for listening to my questions and my requests. Help me to always trust that You will answer in Your time and in the way that is best for me. Amen.

God has told us in His Word that we are to present all of our requests to Him (see Philippians 4:6). David obviously did this (there must be at least one question in every one of David's psalms!), and David also expected God to answer Him. For today, though, we'll take a break from David and his psalms and take a look at what the New Testament has to tell us about requesting things from God. Read Matthew 7:7-11. What did Jesus say we need to do in order to receive what we want (see verses 7-8)?

How is God better than any earthly parent (see verses 9-11)?

According to verse 11, why might we not receive what we ask for?

Read Matthew 6:10 and 1 John 5:14. What is one of the conditions of our receiving what we ask?

According to James 4:3, what is another condition for our requests to be answered positively?

Turn to John 15:7. What other condition did Jesus point out for our requests to be answered?

Because we have faith in Jesus, how are we to approach God with our requests (see 1 John 5:14)?

Read James 5:13-16. What should be our emotional state when we pray and ask something of God?

Right now, stop and ask God in prayer to help you in any area where you feel you need it. Be bold. Don't shrink back. And be confident that God will answer you.

Father, thank You that I can boldly come before You to make requests. Give me confidence to ask for Your help when I need it. I trust You to answer me. Amen.

Day 4 — AVOID THE JOY STEALERS

Lord, I want to be a person who walks through life full of joy, even when the joy stealers try to take it away from me. Help me to stand strong when circumstances try to bring me down. Amen.

One meaning of the word joy is "the emotion evoked by wellbeing, success, or good fortune or by the prospect of possessing what one desires."[1] As Christians, we can expect and hope for the ultimate good life in heaven with God. Unfortunately, we often forget to expect good things—even simple, everyday good things—in *this* world. One reason we miss these things is that we are sidetracked and deceived by joy stealers. In her book *Seven Things That Steal Your Joy*, Joyce Meyer identifies seven joy stealers.[2] Let's look at each of these and then see what the psalms tell us about joy.

Joy Stealer #1: Works of the Flesh

When we expend our energy attempting to do God's job, we allow our joy to be taken away. When we think that everything that happens depends on us and take action, thinking we are in control, we let our joy be stolen.

We need to get to the point where we can be happy without ever having what we want, or we will never receive what we want. God wants us to have abundant lives filled with many blessings, but in order to receive those blessings, we have to put God first and follow His instructions about how we should live. This is no easy task, but if we don't work on this, our joy will be gone!

No matter what our circumstances are, we should always recognize that God is in control, that He knows what He is doing, and that He is deserving of our thanks. Otherwise, we may miss having the blessings and joy that God wants to give us. Read Psalm 51:8-12. What did David want God to do so that his joy would be restored?

_____
_____
_____
_____

Joy Stealer #2: Religious Legalism

Following a strict set of rules of our own making in order to feel righteous in God's eyes will steal joy from us.

As we seek God and walk in the Spirit, God will guide us to follow *His* ways in obedience. It is when we start to think that we can earn God's approval by following rules we make for ourselves that our joy is stolen from us. We must remember that we are made righteous by faith alone. We need to stop having unrealistic religious expectations of ourselves and stop being critical of our efforts to keep "laws" that we made, not ones that God tells us to follow. We need to enjoy God and simply obey His rules for living. Read Psalm 19:7-8. What do God's laws do for us?

_____
_____
_____
_____

Joy Stealer #3: Complicating Simple Issues

We have a tendency to take things that are simple and fun and make them complicated and burdensome. Satan loves to distract us by confusing things and creating complications where they need not exist. He will do whatever he can to prevent us from experiencing God's joy.

We need to learn to live life by being honest with ourselves and with others and simply enjoying the little things in life. We need to stop working so hard and being so busy that we miss the joyful things and people around us. Sometimes we actually think that there's no time for just relaxing or enjoying a good laugh. Read Psalm 65:9-13. Why does all of creation sing for joy, and why should we?

_____
_____
_____
_____

Joy Stealer #4: Excessive Reasoning

Excessive reasoning involves trying to find answers for something that we cannot understand. We continue to ask why something happened or how something came to be instead of simply accepting the fact that there are some things that we cannot comprehend. We should wait on God and trust Him, but instead, we let worry, frustration, resentment and confusion steal our joy! Read Psalm 91:1-2. Why did David trust God, and where did David find rest?

_____
_____
_____
_____

Joy Stealer #5: Ungodly Anger

Anger is one of the ways we let others know that we're not satisfied with something in our lives. Anger itself is not a sin; but when we become angry, we need to pin down the cause of our anger and then we need to deal with it. This is especially important because anger gives Satan a foothold in our lives (see Ephesians 4:27). Read Psalm 37:8-9. Why did David say that we should turn away from anger? What will happen if we don't turn away from it?

_____
_____
_____
_____

Joy Stealer #6: Jealousy and Envy

The last of the Ten Commandments tells us not to "covet . . . anything that belongs to [our] neighbor" (Exodus 20:17). Unfortunately, this commandment is one of the most abused. Desiring something that someone else has—a bigger house, a better car, more money, a sweeter voice—easily leads to the theft of joy. We need to be content with what we have and be thankful. Read Psalm 73:23-26. (Although David did not write this psalm, a leader of one of his choirs did author it.) What did the psalmist say about his desire for earthly things, and why?

_____
_____
_____
_____

Joy Stealer #7: Habitual Discontentment

Because we are human, there are bound to be times when we will be unhappy about something or unhappy with someone. As long as we don't dwell on those times—as long as we move beyond them—we will feel great joy. But we let our joy be stolen from us when unhappiness becomes our way of life. When we are unhappy all of the time, we are not able to be as close to God as we should be, and we are not able to see what God is trying to have us learn. We must enjoy where we are on the way to where we are going. Read Psalm 68:3. How should people who are righteous act?

_____
_____
_____
_____

Dear God, I want to experience all the joy You have for me. Teach me to keep things simple, to be content and to trust You and Your Word. Amen.

PRAISE AND THANK GOD — Day 5

Dear heavenly Father, I want to fill myself with praise for You and thanks to You. I commit to pursuing this with my whole heart! Amen.

It is hard to harbor negative emotions when our hearts are filled with praise and thanksgiving to God for what He has done for us. Lifting our hearts up to God gets us looking in the right direction for the right reasons! For what did David praise and thank God in the following psalms?

Psalm	Things for which David praised and thanked God
7:17	
9:1	
21:13	
28:6-7	
30:11-12	
57:9-10	
68:19	
144:1-2	

David obviously included praise and thanksgiving to God in almost every psalm that he wrote, but Psalm 103 is an entire psalm calling us to praise and thanksgiving. What are some of the reasons for praising God that David gave in this psalm?

_____
_____
_____
_____

Look once more at all of the reasons to praise and thank God that David wrote about. Place an asterisk next to those that have personal meaning for you. Then include your praise and thanks in the prayer below.

> Dear Lord, I praise You and thank You for [list your items]. Help me to develop a lifestyle that includes daily praise and thanksgiving. Thank You for all that You do for me. Guide me with Your Word. Amen.

REFLECTION AND APPLICATION

Day 6

Dear Lord, help me to look at my life honestly so that I can identify the joy stealers Satan is trying to use to lead me astray. I want every day of my life to be filled with Your joy that comes from above. Amen.

Previously, we looked at seven ways Satan uses to try to steal our joy and keep us from living as God wants us to live. Today, take a few minutes to review the descriptions of the joy stealers, and then think about whether any of them have any power over you. Using a scale of 1 to 10 (with 1 indicating no power and 10 being a crushing amount of power), indicate the level of power that each joy stealer has over you. Next to that number, write at least one specific action you will take to send this particular joy stealer out of your life.

Joy stealer	Power	Action
Works of the flesh		
Religious legalism		
Complicating simple issues		
Excessive reasoning		
Ungodly anger		
Jealousy and envy		
Habitual discontentment		

Lord, help me to take action when I feel that my joy is being stolen away. I want every day to be my best day, and I certainly don't want Satan to have his way with my life and how I live. With Your help, I know I can live with joy every day! Amen.

Day 7

REFLECTION AND APPLICATION

Lord, I want to pour out my heart to You just as David did. Help me to follow his example today. Give me the words to express my heart to You. Amen.

Today, it's your turn to follow David's example and be a psalmist! Following the instructions below, write your own personal psalm to God. Make this your rough draft, and then, when you have your ideas together, write it all out on a piece of stationery and keep it in your Bible.

Begin by taking several minutes and pray and think about what you are experiencing right now. Sit and listen to what you hear from your heart. When you're ready, write down your topic: Praise and thanksgiving? A question? A request? Need help with something or someone? Tell what it is about God that makes you think He will hear you/listen to you/answer you.

_____
_____
_____
_____
_____

Now write down how you feel. Sad? Hurting? Joyful? Grateful?

_____
_____
_____
_____

Next, write down who God is to you. What about His character do you love/need/depend on?

_____
_____
_____

Continue by writing down a few things that God has done for you in the past that remind you of how much He loves you and how He only wants the best for you.

_____
_____
_____
_____
_____

Finally, express your belief in God and His power. Praise and thank Him ahead of time for what He is going to do.

_____
_____
_____
_____
_____

Remember that this is a rough draft and you can go back and change any words as you feel called to do (though it's possible that you won't need to change anything!). Also note that style is not that important. The most important thing to remember is that God wants to hear what's on your heart and mind: He's interested in your honesty. When you're finished writing the final draft of your psalm, read your psalm out loud to God. He will be so very glad to hear from you!

> Heavenly Father, I am grateful that You hear my prayers and care about me. Help me to make my thanks to You not just a daily habit but also a through-the-day habit. I have so much for which to praise You. Amen.

Notes

1. *Merriam-Webster's Collegiate Dictionary*, 11th ed., s.v. "joy."
2. Joyce Meyer, *Seven Things That Steal Your Joy: Overcoming the Obstacles to Your Happiness* (NY: Warner Faith, 2004).

Group Prayer Requests

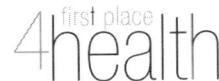

Today's Date: _____

Name	Request

Results

Week Eleven

give your life away

SCRIPTURE MEMORY VERSE
But just as you excel in everything—in faith, in speech, in knowledge, in complete earnestness and in your love for us—see that you also excel in this grace of giving.
2 CORINTHIANS 8:7

"Excel in this grace of giving"—so reads this week's memory verse. But what does giving actually require? Usually when we hear the word "giving" in relation to the Church, we immediately think of giving money—tithing. Certainly the Bible says that we should tithe, or give a tenth of our income to God (see Leviticus 27:30; Numbers 18:26; Deuteronomy 14:22-29). But for Christians, giving involves more than just money.

To excel at giving, we must listen and look for needs that must be filled and then try to fill them. Our hearts should be *ready* to serve, and we must *look for* ways to do so. We must be willing to put others above ourselves. We must be willing to change our schedules at a moment's notice, committing to sacrifice what *we* want to do and trusting in God to extend His strength and wisdom to see us through what needs to be done.

GIVE GENEROUSLY — Day 1

Lord, I want to be a giver, not a taker. I want to be more like You every day, noticing the needs of others and stepping out to serve. Amen.

One of the subjects of Paul's second letter to the Corinthians is the matter of taking up a collection of money for the Christians in Jerusalem who were in need of help. The Corinthians had started (but not finished) a collection, so Paul tells them about the Macedonian churches to provide them with an example of generosity. Read 2 Corinthians 8:1-9, the context of our memory verse. What did God give to the Macedonian churches (see verse 1)?

What was their life like at the time (see verse 2)?

How did these circumstances affect their giving (see verse 2)?

What was their attitude about giving (see verses 2-4)?

What were some of the details about their generosity that were included in verses 3-5?

What about this situation shows that God's grace was abundant in the Macedonian churches?

In what five things did the Corinthians excel, and what sixth thing did Paul want them to add (see verse 7)?

1.
2.
3.
4.
5.
6.

Why did Paul not want to *command* them to give (see verse 8)?

How was Jesus an example of a generous giver (see verse 9)?

Think about your own heart attitude toward giving and the six things in which you can excel. Are there some areas in which you need to improve? Spend time in prayer considering what God wants you to change so that you can excel in the grace of giving in every area of your life.

> *Lord, I want to excel in the grace of giving in every area of my life. Help me to follow Your example. Give me an attitude of overflowing generosity. Amen.*

Day 2

GIVE AS A DAILY HABIT

Lord, I know that a lifestyle of giving is based on daily decisions to be obedient to You. Open my eyes to the ways I can give of myself, and help me to have a daily habit of giving. Thank You, Lord. Amen.

In his book *Today Matters: 12 Daily Practices to Guarantee Tomorrow's Success*, John C. Maxwell talks about the fact that what we do on a daily basis determines how successful we will be in life. One of the 12 ways Maxwell says to be successful is to develop a lifestyle of generosity that involves these four daily habits:

1. Value people: treat everyone with respect.
2. Know what people value: listen to others and seek to understand them.
3. Make yourself more valuable: grow in order to give, as we cannot give what we do not possess.
4. Do things that God values: In the same way that God unconditionally loves people, so must we.[1]

Look at the following four verses, each of which pertains to one of the four habits given above. After you read each verse, indicate the biblical principle that relates to one of Maxwell's suggested daily habits. Then state a specific way you can put the principle into action.

Verse	Biblical principle	Daily action
Matt. 7:12		
Jas. 1:19		
Col. 1:10		
Rom. 12:10		

Another biblical principle about daily giving is described in Hebrews 3:13. What are we supposed to do daily?

What will this help us to do?

Read Romans 12:16. What are we encouraged to do, and why?

Dear heavenly Father, help me to more consciously value all people, even myself. I want to give daily of myself so that I can improve the day of everyone I meet and so that every day can be my best day. Amen.

GIVE FROM YOUR GIFTS

Day 3

Dear God, help me to be willing to give away my talents, my time and my treasure each day. I want to be focused on others and not on myself. Amen.

God has given each of us spiritual gifts and talents. They are part of who we are. When we give from our area of giftedness, we experience the special joy of knowing that we were designed by God to be able to bless others in this way.

Do you know what your spiritual gift is? You may have the gift of mercy—the ability to sit willingly by the bedside of someone who is ill or grieve with a friend who has lost a loved one. You may have the gift of teaching—using your gift to help someone learn a new skill or to coach a sports team. You may have the gift of hospitality—cooking meals to take to a friend who has just had a baby, or having friends over for a meal you provide.

Be creative about using your gifts. Perhaps you love to bake, but you also want to feed your family wisely and not have too many tempting treats around the house. So whenever you bake, you might only keep a small amount of the yummy baked goods, and then take the rest to a friend in need or share with a group you will be attending. What a wonderful, healthy way to give from your gift of hospitality!

There are several verses in the Bible that describe gifts of the Spirit, so if you don't know which gift is yours (and, of course, you may have more than one gift!), read Romans 12:6-8, 1 Corinthians 12:8-10,28, Ephesians 4:11 and 1 Peter 4:11. Which gift(s) of the Spirit do you have?

How are you currently using your gift?

Read 1 Corinthians 14:12. What should we always keep in mind as we think about spiritual gifts?

Now turn to 1 Corinthians 12:4-7. What is the same about all spiritual gifts (see verses 4-5)?

Why are we given spiritual gifts (see verse 7)?

Based on the verses from 1 Corinthians, it is clear that the Holy Spirit determines who gets what gifts. Our part is to use the gift(s) to bless and serve others! But what if we see a need that doesn't fit into our area of giftedness? Should we try to get someone else to do what needs to be done? This might work out, but in many cases, we must give ourselves away, doing good deeds out of sacrifice even when we are not gifted in a particular area. Read 1 Peter 2:12. How should we live?

When people see our good deeds, what will they do?

Lord, You are the giver of gifts. Help me to use whatever gifts You have given to me to bless and serve others. I want my life to shine as a light for You. Amen.

Day 4 — GIVE TO OTHERS FIRST

Lord, thank You for my family and for my friends. Show me ways that I can daily give to them as well as to everyone I meet. Amen.

Everyone in a family needs to be a giver in order for that family to function well. Husbands and wives need to give themselves away to be there for each other. Parents must give themselves away to meet the many needs of their children. As children grow and understand what to do, they also need to be active givers, helping out with family needs as they can, whether it is doing chores or giving hugs. Beyond our families, we need to be ready to help out friends and neighbors. And, as the Bible tells us, there are still others to whom we need to reach out. Read Matthew 25:31-46. When Jesus comes again, into what two groups will He separate everyone?

_____
_____
_____
_____

What are several things that those He saves will have done while on earth (see verses 35-36)?

_____
_____
_____
_____

When we do those things for others, for whom are we really doing them (see verse 40)?

_____
_____
_____

What will happen to people who don't give to others (see verse 46)?

Take a minute or two and think about what you do for "the least of these." What are some areas in which you need to improve? What is at least one specific way you can improve in that area?

According to Luke 6:38, what happens to us when we give?

When was a time when you have seen this principle in action?

Let's finish this day by looking at Acts 20:35. What was Jesus' message about giving?

Lord, help me to remember each day that it is more blessed to give than to receive. Thank You for setting the example for me. Amen.

Day 5

GIVE WITH YOUR WHOLE HEART

Dear heavenly Father, I don't want to be a lukewarm, halfhearted person. Please help me to learn how to be wholehearted in every area of my life. Amen.

There seems to be a lack of wholehearted people in this world. So many people live their daily lives halfheartedly. They are too busy, too tired or just plain too lazy to give their all. Wholehearted living—much less giving—is a rarity! But God has something different in mind. He wants our complete attention, and He wants every bit of every one of us. He wants us to be "all in" when it comes to giving and living. Read Revelation 3:15-16. What does Jesus say about being "lukewarm"?

Turn to Deuteronomy 4:29. How are we to find God?

Wholehearted giving starts with wholehearted seeking! God wants us to have a heart that is single-mindedly focused on Him. Read Colossians 3:23-24. In what way are we to do anything?

How do you think this attitude lends itself to giving with your whole heart?

Turn to Matthew 22:34-39. In what three ways are we to love God (see verse 37)?

1.
2.
3.

Think about how you love God. For each of the ways listed above, what is one specific thing you do to show God that you love Him in that way?

1.
2.
3.

When we love the Lord wholeheartedly, we are ready and willing to give ourselves away! Read 2 Corinthians 9:7-11. How does God expect us to give (see verse 7)?

How does God help us do what He wants (see verses 8-11)?

What will happen as a result of our giving (see verse 11)?

_____
_____
_____
_____

Dear Lord, I love You with all my heart, soul and mind. Show me how to love my neighbor as myself, living a wholehearted life of giving cheerfully. Amen.

Day 6 — REFLECTION AND APPLICATION

Lord, I want to excel in everything, especially in giving of myself to others. Guide me to see how I am doing in this area of my life. Amen.

Today, let's focus on giving to others and assess our giving quotient. How well are you doing in the area of giving to others? Are there some things that come easily for you and other things that are difficult? Are some things so daunting that you haven't tried yet to do them? In the chart below, for each of the people listed, note how you are doing, tell what if anything is holding you back, and think of at least one specific action you can take to improve in that area of giving.

Area of giving	How I'm doing	What's holding me back	Action I need to take
Spouse			
Children			
Parents			

Area of giving	How I'm doing	What's holding me back	Action I need to take
Other family			
Friends			
Neighbors			
The hungry and thirsty			
Those who need clothes			
The sick			
Prisoners			
Others			

Almighty God, I want my giving quotient in regard to others to be growing every day. Help me to overcome any obstacles that hold me back, and give me the wisdom and strength to put improvements into place. Amen.

Day 7

REFLECTION AND APPLICATION

Lord, open my mind to understand and my heart to do the work You have set before me in all areas of giving. Teach me to be the kind of giver You want.

Yesterday, you focused on assessing your giving quotient in regard to others. Today, let's focus on how you're doing in regard to other areas of giving and your attitude. Do you tithe? Do you give just to your church, or does part of your tithe go to charitable organizations that do God's work? How are you using your spiritual gift(s)? Do you give away any of your time (sit with a sick person, read to someone in a nursing home, run errands or do chores for someone who needs the help)? Is your attitude always one that reflects the love You have for God? Are you always a cheerful giver? Do you make it a point to encourage others?

In the chart below, for each type of giving, note how you are doing, tell what if anything is holding you back, and think of at least one specific action you can take to improve that type of giving.

Type of giving	How I'm doing	What's holding me back	Action I need to take
Tithing			
Use of spiritual gift(s)			
Time			

Type of giving	How I'm doing	What's holding me back	Action I need to take
Attitude that shows God's love			
Attitude that is cheerful			
Encouragement			

As you fill in the chart, seek God's help for any answers that elude you. If there seem to be situations in your life that could make giving in some of these areas impossible, ask God to show you a way to give that won't overtax you or overburden your finances. Put yourself in God's capable hands, and watch Him work in your life!

> *Thank You, Lord, for helping me to see where I need to make improvements in the types of giving I should be doing and in the attitude I should have as I give. Help me to never stop trying to make every day the best day. Amen.*

Note
1. John C. Maxwell, *Today Matters: 12 Daily Practices to Guarantee Tomorrow's Success* (NY: Warner Faith, 2005), p. 247.

Group Prayer Requests

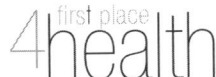

Today's Date: _____

Name	Request

Results

_____
_____
_____
_____
_____

Week Twelve

time to celebrate!

To help shape your brief victory celebration testimony, work through the following questions in your prayer journal:

Day One: List some of the benefits you have gained by allowing the Lord to transform your life through this 12-week First Place 4 Health session. Be sure to list benefits you have received in the physical, mental, emotional and spiritual realms of your being.

Day Two: In what ways have you most significantly changed *mentally*? Have you seen a shift in the ways you think about yourself, food, your relationships or God? How has Scripture memory been a part of these shifts?

Day Three: In what ways have you most significantly changed *emotionally*? Have you begun to identify how your feelings influence your relationship to food and exercise? What are you doing to stay aware of your emotions, both positive and negative?

Day Four: In what ways have you most significantly changed *spiritually*? How has your relationship with God deepened? How has drawing closer to Him made a difference in the other three areas of your life?

Day Five: In what ways have you most significantly changed *physically*? Have you met or exceeded your weight/measurement goals? How has your health improved the past 12 weeks?

Day Six: Was there one person in your First Place 4 Health group who was particularly encouraging to you? How did their kindness make a difference in your First Place 4 Health journey?

Day Seven: Summarize the previous six questions into a one-page testimony, or "faith story," to share at your group's victory celebration.

May our gracious Lord bless and keep you as you continue to keep Him first in all things!

Make Every Day Your Best Day
leader discussion guide

For in-depth information, guidance and helpful tips about leading a successful First Place 4 Health group, spend time studying the *First Place 4 Health Leader's Guide*. In it, you will find valuable answers to most of your questions, as well as personal insights from many First Place 4 Health group leaders.

For the group meetings in this session, be sure to read and consider each week's discussion topics several days before the meeting—some questions and activities require supplies and/or planning to complete. Also, if you are leading a large group, plan to break into smaller groups for discussion and then come together as a large group to share your answers and responses. Make sure to appoint a capable leader for each small group so that discussions stay focused and on track (and be sure each group records their answers!).

week one: welcome to *Make Every Day Your Best Day*
During this first week, welcome the members to your group, provide a brief overview of the First Place 4 Health program, explain what is expected of the participants at each of the weekly meetings, and collect the Member Surveys. (See the *First Place 4 Health Leader's Guide* for a detailed outline of how to conduct the first week's meeting.)

week two: leave yesterday behind
If possible, bring a bottle of water for each group member (or ahead of time, ask each of them to bring his or her own water bottle). Take a moment to drink some water together and commit to drinking more water, making it a healthy habit.

Make sure that everyone understands that "in Christ" means more than just understanding who Jesus is (see Day 1). It also means being united to Jesus so that we are transformed, or made new.

Have someone read aloud Psalm 118:24 (see Day 2). Ask for volunteers to share one reason they can rejoice in today. Lead a discussion about how easy and/or hard it is to rejoice on any given day. Encourage honest, transparent sharing, setting the tone for appropriate openness in your group.

Have each participant write down on a small strip of paper one or more things that they have felt guilty about in the past (see Day 3). Have them crumple up the paper and, as they hold it, remind them that when they accepted Jesus as their Savior, their sins were forgiven. Decide on an appropriate way to dispose of the papers (if possible, go outside to a fire pit and burn them while the group watches) and assure the study group that the things they wrote down are now in God's sea of forgetfulness. They can leave the past behind.

Talk about the way the world is today and how everything seems to change so fast (see Day 4). Share a little bit about how generally in the past people lived at a slower pace but how technology in particular has brought—and continues to bring—a great deal of change to our world. Ask volunteers to share how our changeable world contrasts with God's unchanging character. Consider how powerful our God is in that He is the same yesterday, today and forever. Optional: If you have time, invite volunteers to share stories of recent changes in their lives and how God has worked to grow them as they have walked through the changes.

Have a volunteer read aloud Romans 8:28 (see Day 5). Then invite other volunteers to share what they think this Scripture means and how they have experienced it in their lives. Help the group see how God unfolds His purpose even through hard times.

Spend some time talking about the importance of drinking water (see Day 6). Emphasize the need to stay hydrated during exercise and especially during hot weather and at high altitudes. Encourage group members to pass on the water-drinking habit to the rest of their families.

Challenge the group to notice how drinking water makes a difference in their lives.

Talk about vision statements (see Day 7). Make sure the group members understand that creating each of their visions for a healthy future is a process; they can start now (by using the guided thoughts provided in the study, if they want) and then continue to develop the vision in the days ahead. Invite volunteers to share parts of their vision statements with the group as examples. Share your vision statement with them as well. It will help them get to know you and set the pace for them to be faithful to do it.

week three: let tomorrow take care of itself

Discuss with your group the types of cares we can give to God (see Day 1). Encourage each group member to keep in their personal journal a brief description of the cares and worries that they have given to God, noting how God has sustained them and how God has taken care of their concerns. If there is time, ask a volunteer to read aloud Matthew 6:25-32, and then discuss what Jesus had to say about worrying.

Lead a discussion about some of the modern "chariots and horses" that people trust in today (see Day 2). Talk about why trust in any earthly thing is not nearly as reliable as trusting in God. Ask volunteers to share some of the specific steps that can be taken so that trust in God will be the first thing that comes to mind in worrisome situations.

Discuss why presenting our requests to God is an important part of an abundant life (see Day 3). Ask a volunteer to share briefly a story about having done this and then being blessed with "the peace of God." Ask other volunteers to share the sorts of thoughts that should be our focus and whether or not such thoughts are always possible.

Discuss the difference between our being in control of our lives and God's being in control (see Day 4). Ask a volunteer to share a brief story about a time when he or she felt controlled by the Spirit. Make sure that the group understands the point of Psalm 37:23-24—our obedience is a requirement for God to bless us.

Ask someone to read aloud Psalm 121, emphasizing the words "watch" and "watches" (see Day 5). Ask for volunteers to tell what God watches over, when He watches and what God does as He watches over us. Invite volunteers to tell what it feels like to know that God is watching us all of the time.

Ask volunteers to share specific steps we can take to handle worry better (see Day 6). After inviting the group members to take a few deep breaths, play the song "Breathe" in class (see Day 7). While you all listen to the music, have everyone close their eyes and practice the deep-breathing technique mentioned in the text.

week four: have the right attitude

Discuss Psalm 31 and why our attitudes should be the same as David's was (see Day 1). Talk about how various things—time pressure, for instance—affect our attitudes. Talk about good, bad and ugly attitudes and encourage the group members to share their ideas for specific steps to take to renew their minds.

Ask for volunteers to tell how God and hope are related (see Day 2). Stress the point that because of God's unfailing love, we always have hope and we can be joyful and praise God for the promises He keeps. Ask for volunteers to briefly tell about times when God worked in their lives to give them hope, even when they were downcast.

Ask for volunteers to suggest reasons why most people are harder on themselves than on others (see Day 3). Discuss the story about the boy who was healed, emphasizing that the faith of the boy's father is similar to our own because our faith is not perfect, but we want it to be perfect and that's what we strive for it to be. Invite volunteers to tell why prayer bolsters belief.

Discuss the attitude of compassion that Jesus had and how we can reflect that same attitude (see Day 4). Go over with the group what the "clothes" we should have on look like in practical terms (see Colossians 3:12-14). Ask if anyone has a story about "building up" someone else that they would like to share to encourage everyone.

Read Psalm 100 out loud (see Day 5). Talk about the connection between joy and thankfulness. Have each member of the class share one thing they are thankful for and why that gives them joy. Share creative ideas for building the habit of thankfulness and joy into our everyday lives.

Invite volunteers to share one nugget of truth they learned this week and the specific step they will take to implement that truth in their lives (see Day 6). Perhaps even set up a plan of action for accountability, if the group members appear interested in doing that.

Ask a few group members to list some of the items that they placed on their "thankfulness list" (see Day 7). Ask how this exercise of intentionally looking for the blessings that God gives to us each day affected their attitude during the week. Discuss some of the ways that the group can continue to develop a lifestyle of praise and worship. Spend time in prayer asking God to work on attitudes and for God to increase the level of hope in the lives of everyone in the group.

week five: make wise decisions one day at a time

Lead a discussion about the difference between wisdom and understanding, and how both relate to "the fear of the Lord" (see Day 1). Make sure that everyone understands that "fear of the Lord" does not mean being scared of God, but it does mean having a healthy respect for how powerful God is.

Discuss what James has to say about wisdom, especially how we show that we have wisdom (see Day 2). Ask volunteers to suggest some dos and don'ts of decision making and how to seek God's wisdom when making decisions. Encourage the group members to make a commitment to "shine like stars," as Daniel did.

Briefly review how Solomon became wise, and ask a volunteer to recap the story about the two women who claimed the same baby (see Day 3). With the group, discuss the difference between Solomon's early decisions and his later ones and how God reacted to the change.

Ask volunteers to tell where people usually go for advice or what people often consult when important decisions have to be made (see Day 4).

Then ask other volunteers to tell where the Bible tells us we should go for advice and why. Lead a discussion on the disadvantages of using earthly resources and the advantages of using those provided by God.

Invite volunteers to suggest which decisions are the most important in life (see Day 5). Remind the group that *the* most important decision is belief in Jesus, which leads to eternal life. Mention that anyone who has questions about becoming a Christian or anyone who has prayed the prayer in the study is welcome to come to you and chat after the meeting.

Invite volunteers to share the experiences they had when they tried to start conversations about wisdom (see Day 6). See if anyone was able to have a spiritual conversation with someone. Also ask volunteers to tell how people can quietly shine wisdom.

Talk to the class about the importance of physical fitness (see Day 7). Remind the group that being physically active is an important part of the First Place 4 Health program. Ask volunteers to share their action plans for physical fitness, and talk about the many options that are available for consideration. Urge them to make their fitness decision and take action today!

week six: take small steps in the right direction

Share a story about a "baby step" that you have taken recently (see Day 1). Set the tone that baby steps are a great thing, and encourage a few volunteers to share stories about baby steps they have taken. Encourage your group members to be excited like a little child about the baby steps they are taking.

Ask for volunteers to tell reasons why slow steady steps are valuable (see Day 2). Focus on the attribute of patience, and point out that it takes the Holy Spirit to grow this fruit in us. Invite volunteers to give their ideas about how we "keep in step" with the Holy Spirit.

Focus a discussion on 2 Corinthians 12:9-10, and make sure that everyone understands that God's power can most easily be displayed when we are weak (see Day 3). Invite volunteers to share why depending "on flesh" for strength is not a good idea (Jeremiah 17:5) and how God's power can strengthen us when we are weak.

Invite a few group members to share some of the steep climbs that many people experience in life (see Day 4). Discuss the importance of preparing mentally and physically for the climbs of life. Ask volunteers to share specific ways we can align our thoughts with Christ and depend on God for our safety.

If anyone in your group is a runner, ask him or her to tell what they do to prepare to run (see Day 5). Ask volunteers to tell why we can look to God for help as we run the race of life—why is God able to understand what we go through.

Invite the group members to suggest ways other than those mentioned in the text that will give us a slight edge as we take steps in the right direction (see Day 6).

Discuss the concept of safety and how it applies in different areas of our lives—emotionally, spiritually, mentally and physically (see Day 7). Invite group members to tell some of the things that make them feel safe.

week seven: watch out for the father of lies

Lead a discussion about the deceptions Satan uses to try to turn us to his dark ways (see Day 1). Invite one or two volunteers to briefly share a story about breaking free to the truth after a time of deception.

Ask volunteers to tell some ideas the world has about beauty and to tell what happens to earthly beauty (see Day 2). Focus on the deceptions about beauty that society would have us believe. Then emphasize God's love for us and His concern about our inner beauty. Invite volunteers to tell how inner beauty is seen outwardly.

Ask volunteers to describe ways that Satan tries to "devour" us (see Day 3; 1 Peter 5:8). Invite someone to explain how we can resist the devil. Make sure that the group members understand that Scripture can be used as a powerful weapon in spiritual warfare, and that's one of the reasons it's an important part of the First Place 4 Health program. Also review how God helps us whenever we're tempted to do wrong.

Discuss the power of prayer (see Day 4). Review David's requests and comments in Psalm 86. Urge your group members to practice this type of praying so that they can establish more "prayer power" in their lives.

Invite volunteers to tell some specific ways that Satan masquerades as "an angel of light" (see Day 5). Ask other volunteers to tell specific ways that we can make our "light shine before men" (Matthew 5:16).

Briefly review the fact that God's ways—His thoughts, His actions, His love, His everything—are beyond our human capacity to understand (see Day 6). Emphasize that as un-understandable as God is, one day we *will* understand and see Him in person!

Invite volunteers to tell different specific ways that group members can encourage other people (see Day 7). Make sure that verbal and non-verbal ways of encouragement are mentioned.

week eight: get your spiritual life in shape

Ask for volunteers to tell the four conditions we must meet in order to "draw near to God" (see Day 1; Hebrews 10:22). Invite other volunteers to tell some of the practical ways we hold on to hope and how this affects our lives. Make clear that as we draw closer to God, He draws increasingly closer to us.

Call for volunteers to tell why prayer is so important, no matter what our circumstances or situations (see Day 2). Ask if anyone is willing to share a brief story about answered prayer, even if the answer was no.

Invite volunteers to tell some of the benefits of reading the Bible, as described in Psalm 119 (see Day 3).

Ask the group members to list the various ways of worship that the Bible mentions (see Day 4). Invite volunteers to rate their comfort level with the various forms. Make clear to the group members that comfort level does not determine whether one form of worship is better than another. Stress the fact that God wants to see worship that is done "in spirit and in truth"—that is what determines whether something is worship in God's eyes (John 4:23).

Lead a discussion about the importance and value of Christian fellowship (see Day 5). Ask for volunteers to explain why fellowship is an encouragement for all those who take part in it.

Invite volunteers to share with the group one thing they learned from one of the memory verses from this study (see Day 6).

Ask volunteers to tell specific ways that worship can be incorporated into our everyday lives (see Day 7). Then invite volunteers to share the new way they will try or have already tried, and how they feel about it.

If there is time, play two or three worship songs that reflect different musical styles, and provide word sheets for each song. As the group listens to each song, invite them to sing along and worship!

week nine: take care of your physical health

Discuss the contrast between physical training and godliness (see Day 1). Ask volunteers to explain how we reveal what we have stored in our hearts. Invite other volunteers to tell specific ways that we can guard our hearts.

Invite volunteers to tell what sort of strength is needed for each area of our lives—physical, spiritual, mental and emotional (see Day 2). Ask if anyone is comfortable to share which area he or she needs to work on most to gain more strength.

Invite the group members to give some real-life situations in which flexibility would be necessary (see Day 3). Ask for a volunteer to explain how Mary appeared to be more flexible than Martha, and ask someone else to explain what the ultimate goal of our flexibility is.

Invite someone to tell what our purpose should be no matter what we do, and invite someone else to explain how this relates to the food we eat (see Day 4). Ask volunteers to explain why we should regard our bodies as temples and, therefore, also be mindful of what goes into them. Also ask someone to explain how what we eat may influence other people.

Ask for volunteers to explain the importance of rest to both our bodies and to our souls (see Day 5). Talk about both the commandment God gave to us and the example Jesus set for us.

Ask volunteers to share some of the specific ways that they came up with for putting into practice improvements to guard and strengthen their hearts (see Day 6).

Talk in general about the need to physically rest and the need to spend time resting in and with God (see Day 7). Ask the group members for practical suggestions for how to get the rest we need.

week ten: guard your heart and emotions daily

Invite volunteers to describe the way David shares his heart and emotions with God (see Day 1). Ask for volunteers to explain why hope is like an anchor and how God guarantees our safety.

Lead a discussion about being honest with God and why "honesty is the best policy" (see Day 2). Ask group members to think of the most honest person they know and to describe the qualities of that person that are attractive and how they know that the person is honest. Briefly discuss the world's view of dishonest people and what does or does not happen to dishonest people.

Ask volunteers to tell why God doesn't always answer our prayers the way we want or expect (see Day 3). Invite the group members to go over the conditions that are necessary for our requests to be answered. Invite anyone willing to briefly share a story of how God answered one of his or her prayers.

Share with the group which of the seven joy stealers is the one that you have the most trouble fighting and what you have learned that helps you have victory over the joy stealers (see Day 4). Invite a few other group members to briefly share their experiences so that everyone can learn more ways to keep their joy alive.

Go around the group and ask each member to tell one thing for which he or she can praise and thank God (see Day 5). If you have time, go around the group a couple of times. Invite volunteers to explain why praising and thanking God, especially during difficult circumstances, is a way to call on God and to dispel negative thoughts and feelings.

Have everyone take out their joy-stealer chart, and invite volunteers to share the action and the Scripture they plan to use to fight one of the joy stealers (see Day 6). Ask if anyone is willing to read aloud the psalm they wrote (see Day 7). Everyone will be blessed if some step up to do this!

week eleven: give your life away

Briefly review the circumstances of the Macedonian churches during the time of Paul's letter to the Corinthians (see Day 1). Ask someone to explain how the Macedonian churches were able to give joyfully, even though they were living a life with many trials. Ask for opinions about how this compares to the way giving often happens today.

Discuss John Maxwell's ideas for daily generosity (see Day 2). Ask volunteers to tell which of the daily habits are easiest for them and which are the hardest. Invite suggestions for actions to take in order to improve in each area.

Ask the group if everyone has determined which gifts of the Spirit they have (see Day 3). Ask the group to suggest different and creative ways to use some of the gifts to help other members see the possibilities they may not have thought of. Call on the group members to explain how sacrifice is required when we give from our gifts.

Ask volunteers to describe the differences between sheep and goats as Jesus described them (see Day 4). Invite volunteers to suggest ways that we can give to "the least of these."

Have a volunteer read aloud Colossians 3:23-24 (see Day 5). Ask for volunteers to tell what daily action shows their love of God. Invite other volunteers to describe the difference between what wholehearted giving and halfhearted (or lukewarm) giving looks like. Ask volunteers to share where in their lives they are practicing wholehearted giving and where they are only giving halfheartedly and want to do a better job.

Discuss the fact that giving in every area of our lives is not easy to do, and ask if anyone was able to write that he or she does well in every area listed in the chart (see Day 6). Briefly go over each area of giving and discuss in general terms what may hold people back from giving wholeheartedly in each area. Ask volunteers to tell specific ways that they plan to act in order to make improvements where necessary.

Talk about the various types of giving that God expects of us (see Day 7). Briefly go over each type of giving and discuss in general terms why giving that way wholeheartedly may be difficult. Ask volunteers to share any struggles they have and discuss specific ways they plan to act in order to make improvements where necessary.

week twelve: time to celebrate!

Even though most of your meeting this week will be a victory celebration, take some time at the beginning of the meeting to talk about how much God loves each person in the group and how each of us is called to love our brothers and sisters in Christ. (See "Planning a Victory Celebration" in the *First Place 4 Health Leader's Guide* for ideas about throwing a successful celebration for your group.)

For the rest of the study time, allow each member to tell his or her *Make Every Day Your Best Day* story. Give members an equal opportunity to share the goals they set for themselves at the beginning of the session and talk about the challenges and good things God has done for them throughout the process. Don't allow the more talkative group members to monopolize all the time. Even the quiet members need an opportunity to share their stories and successes! Even those who have not met their goals have still been part of the journey, so allow them to share and talk about why they did not succeed.

Making a commitment to continue in First Place 4 Health is an important part of victory. Be sure to talk about your group's future plans, and make each person feel welcome to continue to journey with you. End the study by inviting the group to proclaim together Hebrews 12:1-3.

First Place 4 Health menu plans

Each menu plan is based on approximately 1,400 to 1,500 calories per day. All recipe and menu exchanges were determined using the Master-Cook software, a program that accesses a database containing more than 6,000 food items prepared using the United States Department of Agriculture (USDA) publications and information from food manufacturers. As with any nutritional program, MasterCook calculates the nutritional values of the recipes based on ingredients. Nutrition may vary due to how the food is prepared, where the food comes from, soil content, season, ripeness, processing and method of preparation. For these reasons, please use the recipes and menu plans as approximate guides. Consult a physician and/or a registered dietitian before starting a weight-loss program.

For those who need more calories, add the following to the 1,400-calorie plan:

- 1,800 calories: 2 ounce equivalent of meat, 3 ounce equivalent of bread, ½ cup vegetable serving, 1 tsp. fat
- 2,000 calories: 2 ounce equivalent of meat, 4 ounce equivalent of bread, ½ cup vegetable serving, 3 tsp. fat
- 2,200 calories: 2 ounce equivalent of meat, 5 ounce equivalent of bread, ½ cup vegetable serving, ½ cup fruit serving, 5 tsp. fat
- 2,400 calories: 2 ounce equivalent of meat, 6 ounce equivalent of bread, 1 cup vegetable serving, ½ cup fruit serving, 6 tsp. fat

First Week Grocery List

Produce
- [ ] apples
- [ ] asparagus
- [ ] avocados
- [ ] baby spinach
- [ ] bananas
- [ ] basil
- [ ] broccoli florets
- [ ] cantaloupe
- [ ] cherry tomatoes
- [ ] chipotle chiles
- [ ] cilantro
- [ ] cremini mushrooms
- [ ] cucumbers
- [ ] dill
- [ ] English cucumber
- [ ] garlic cloves
- [ ] golden raisins
- [ ] Granny Smith apple
- [ ] green beans
- [ ] green onions
- [ ] green-leaf lettuce
- [ ] lemons
- [ ] limes
- [ ] mint or tarragon
- [ ] onions
- [ ] oranges
- [ ] parsley
- [ ] radishes
- [ ] red onions
- [ ] red potatoes
- [ ] romaine lettuce
- [ ] salad greens, mixed
- [ ] shallots
- [ ] strawberries
- [ ] sugar snap peas
- [ ] thyme
- [ ] tomatoes
- [ ] watercress

Baking/Cooking Products
- [ ] baking powder
- [ ] brown sugar
- [ ] butter
- [ ] canola oil
- [ ] chocolate chips, semisweet
- [ ] flour, all-purpose
- [ ] nonstick cooking spray
- [ ] olive oil, extra-virgin
- [ ] sugar
- [ ] vanilla extract

Spices
- [ ] black pepper
- [ ] cinnamon
- [ ] cumin
- [ ] nutmeg
- [ ] paprika
- [ ] red pepper
- [ ] salt

Nuts/Seeds
- [ ] almonds
- [ ] pecans

Condiments, Spreads and Sauces
- [ ] Dijon mustard
- [ ] honey
- [ ] hummus, plain or flavored
- [ ] margarine, light
- [ ] marinara sauce, lower-sodium
- [ ] salsa
- [ ] soy sauce, lower-sodium
- [ ] taco seasoning

Breads, Cereals and Pasta
- [ ] baked tortilla chips
- [ ] brown rice (such as Uncle Ben's®)
- [ ] corn tortillas
- [ ] dinner rolls, whole-wheat
- [ ] English muffin
- [ ] fettuccine
- [ ] French bread baguette
- [ ] oatmeal
- [ ] oats
- [ ] panko (Japanese breadcrumbs)
- [ ] pita chips, multigrain
- [ ] pitas, whole-wheat
- [ ] puffed rice cereal
- [ ] rigatoni

Canned/Frozen Foods
- [ ] black beans, organic
- [ ] blackberries
- [ ] blueberries
- [ ] chicken broth, fat-free, lower-sodium
- [ ] corn, whole-kernel
- [ ] jalapeno peppers

Dairy Products
- [ ] buttermilk, nonfat
- [ ] cheddar cheese
- [ ] cream cheese, less-fat
- [ ] feta cheese
- [ ] Greek yogurt, 2% reduced-fat
- [ ] heavy whipping cream
- [ ] milk, nonfat
- [ ] Parmesan cheese
- [ ] processed American cheese, light (such as Velveeta Light®)
- [ ] queso fresco
- [ ] vanilla yogurt, lowfat

Juices
- [ ] lemon juice
- [ ] lime juice
- [ ] orange juice

Meat and Poultry
- [ ] bacon
- [ ] chicken breasts
- [ ] eggs
- [ ] flank steak
- [ ] ground beef
- [ ] ground sirloin
- [ ] pork shoulder (Boston butt)
- [ ] pork tenderloin
- [ ] rotisserie chicken
- [ ] rotisserie chicken breast
- [ ] shrimp
- [ ] trout fillets

Miscellaneous
- [ ] instant coffee

First Week Meals and Recipes

DAY 1

Breakfast

Start-the-Day Oatmeal

2 cups nonfat milk	½ tsp. vanilla extract
2 cups oats, regular	½ tsp. cinnamon, ground
½ cup golden raisins	6 tbsp. almonds, sliced and toasted
2 tbsp. honey	
½ tsp. salt	2 tbsp. brown sugar

Bring milk to a boil over medium heat. Stir in oats; cook 5 minutes. Remove from heat; stir in raisins, honey, salt, vanilla and cinnamon. Serve with nuts and sugar. Serves 4.

Nutritional Information: 355 calories; 6.2g fat; 13g protein; 66.3g carbohydrate; 6.1g dietary fiber; 5mg cholesterol; 304mg sodium.

Lunch

Chicken Salad with Avocado

2 tbsp. extra-virgin olive oil	2 cups rotisserie chicken breast, shredded, skinless and boneless
2 tbsp. fresh lime juice	
½ tsp. salt	¾ cup fresh salsa, refrigerated
½ tsp. black pepper, freshly ground	1 ripe avocado, peeled and chopped
¼ cup fresh cilantro, chopped	3 oz. baked tortilla chips

Combine oil, lemon juice, salt and pepper in a medium bowl; stir with a whisk. Add chicken and cilantro; toss to combine. Gently fold in salsa and avocado. Serve with chips. Serves 4.

Nutritional Information: 345 calories; 21g fat; 19.2g protein; 20.4g carbohydrate; 4.5g dietary fiber; 50mg cholesterol; 579mg sodium.

Dinner

Fettuccine with Meatballs

9 oz. fettuccine, refrigerated	½ cup panko (Japanese breadcrumbs)
12 oz. ground beef	⅓ cup fresh basil, chopped

2 garlic cloves, minced
⅜ tsp. salt
¼ tsp. black pepper
1 large egg, lightly beaten
2 tsp. extra-virgin olive oil

1¾ cups lower-sodium marinara sauce
⅓ cup water
1 oz. Parmesan cheese, grated

Cook the pasta according to package directions. Drain and set aside. While the pasta cooks, combine beef, panko, basil, garlic, salt, pepper and egg; shape mixture into 16 meatballs. Heat olive oil in a large skillet over medium-high heat. Add meatballs; cook 5 minutes, browning on all sides. Reduce heat to medium-low. Add marinara and ⅓ cup water. Cover and cook 11 minutes or until meatballs are done. Divide the pasta evenly among 4 plates; top evenly with sauce, meatballs and cheese. Serves 4.

Nutritional Information: 489 calories; 16g fat; 29.1g protein; 71.6g carbohydrate; 2.6g dietary fiber; 147mg cholesterol; 688mg sodium.

DAY 2

Breakfast

Mocha Muffins
⅔ cup nonfat milk
5 tbsp. butter, melted
3 tbsp. instant coffee granules
1½ tsp. vanilla extract
1 large egg, lightly beaten
2 cups all-purpose flour

⅔ cup sugar
½ cup semisweet chocolate chips
2 tsp. baking powder
¼ tsp. salt
nonstick cooking spray

Preheat oven to 400° F. In small bowl, combine milk, butter, coffee granules, vanilla and egg. Set aside. Lightly spoon flour into dry measuring cups; level with a knife. In a large bowl, combine flour, sugar, baking powder and salt; stir well with a whisk. Make a well in the center of the flour mixture. Add milk mixture to flour mixture; stir just until moist. Spoon batter into 12 muffin cups coated with nonstick cooking spray. Bake at 400° F for 18 minutes or until done. Remove muffins from pan immediately; place on a wire rack. Serves 12.

Nutritional Information: 191 calories; 6g fat; 3.6g protein; 32.9g carbohydrate; 1g dietary fiber; 29mg cholesterol; 163mg sodium.

Lunch

Veggie Hummus Pitas

1 (8-oz.) container plain or flavored hummus
4 (6-inch) whole-wheat pitas, halved
4 green-leaf lettuce leaves, halved
¾ cup radishes, thinly sliced
1¼ cups English cucumber, thinly sliced
⅓ cup red onion, thinly sliced
½ cup feta cheese, crumbled
dash of black pepper, freshly ground

Divide hummus mixture evenly among 8 pita halves (about 1½ tablespoons each). Divide lettuce, cucumber, radishes, onion and cheese evenly and stuff into pita halves. Sprinkle with pepper. Serves 4.

Nutritional Information: 344 calories; 14.9g fat; 13.1g protein; 47.1g carbohydrate; 7.7g dietary fiber; 13mg cholesterol; 758mg sodium.

Dinner

Roasted Pork Tenderloin

½ tsp. salt
½ tsp. black pepper, freshly ground
1 lb. pork tenderloin
1 tbsp. extra-virgin olive oil

Sprinkle salt and freshly ground black pepper over pork tenderloin. Heat a large skillet over medium-high heat. Add olive oil to pan; swirl to coat. Add pork to pan; cook 3 minutes, browning on all sides. Bake pork at 400° F for 17 minutes or until a thermometer registers 145° F. Let stand 10 minutes; cut across the grain into thin slices. Serves 4.

Nutritional Information: 170 calories; 7.5g fat; 24g protein; 0.1g carbohydrate; 0.0g dietary fiber; 67mg cholesterol; 338mg sodium.

Fresh Steamed Sugar Snap Peas

3 cups fresh sugar snap peas
1 tbsp. fresh mint or tarragon, chopped
1 tbsp. butter
⅛ tsp. salt
⅛ tsp. black pepper, freshly ground

Steam peas for 5 minutes or until crisp-tender; drain. Combine peas, mint, butter, salt and pepper; toss well. Serve immediately. Serves 4.

Nutritional Information: 46 calories; 3g fat; 1.4g protein; 3.7g carbohydrate; 1.3g dietary fiber; 8mg cholesterol; 96mg sodium.

DAY 3

Breakfast

½ cup oatmeal with ½ tsp. light margarine, dash of nutmeg, dash of cinnamon and ½ apple sliced on top
1 cup nonfat milk

Nutritional Information: 290 calories; 4g fat; 15g protein; 50g carbohydrate; 6g dietary fiber; 4mg cholesterol; 151mg sodium.

Lunch

Sautéed Shrimp and Salad

1 tsp. lemon rind, grated
⅓ cup fresh lemon juice
¼ cup fresh basil, chopped
1½ tsp. paprika
½ tsp. salt
¼ tsp. red pepper, crushed
¼ tsp. black pepper
3 garlic cloves, minced
4 tbsp. extra-virgin olive oil, divided
1 lb. large shrimp, peeled and deveined
2 cups (1-inch) cut asparagus
7 cups romaine lettuce, torn
1 cup watercress, trimmed

Combine lemon rind, juice, basil, paprika, salt, peppers and garlic in small bowl. Whisk in 3 tablespoons oil. Set juice mixture aside. Heat remaining 1 tablespoon oil in a large skillet over medium-high heat. Add shrimp; cook 2 minutes. Add juice mixture; cook 1 minute. Stir in asparagus. Place romaine in a large bowl; toss with shrimp mixture. Divide salad among 4 plates; top each with ¼ cup watercress. Serves 4.

Nutritional Information: 281 calories; 16g fat; 26.2g protein; 9.8g carbohydrate; 3.8g dietary fiber; 172mg cholesterol; 476mg sodium.

Wheat Rolls with Orange Honey Butter

2 tsp. butter, softened
1 tsp. honey
½ tsp. orange rind, grated
4 (1-oz.) whole-wheat dinner rolls

Heat dinner rolls as directed. Combine butter, honey and rind; stir well. Serve each roll with about ½ teaspoon butter mixture. Serves 4.

Nutritional Information: 98 calories; 3.3g fat; 2.5g protein; 16g carbohydrate; 2.2g dietary fiber; 5mg cholesterol; 136mg sodium.

Dinner

Broccoli Rice Casserole with Chicken

3 cups small broccoli florets
1 (8.8-oz.) pouch precooked brown rice (such as Uncle Ben's®)
1 tbsp. extra-virgin olive oil
8 oz. skinless, boneless chicken breasts, cut into bite-size pieces
¼ tsp. salt
½ tsp. black pepper
½ cup green onions, chopped
3 oz. processed American cheese, light, cut into 1-inch pieces
2 tbsp. almonds, sliced and toasted

Steam broccoli for 5 minutes or until crisp-tender; drain and set aside. Heat rice according to package directions. Set aside. Heat oil in a large nonstick skillet over medium-high heat. Add chicken; sprinkle with salt and pepper. Cook for 4 minutes or until done, stirring occasionally. Add onions and cheese, stirring until cheese begins to melt. Stir in rice; fold in broccoli. Cook 1 minute or until thoroughly heated. Sprinkle with almonds. Serves 3.

Nutritional Information: 366 calories; 13g fat; 28.9g protein; 33.7g carbohydrate; 4.5g dietary fiber; 56mg cholesterol; 688mg sodium.

DAY 4

Breakfast

Greek Yogurt with Berry Sauce

⅔ cup blueberries, frozen
⅔ cup blackberries, frozen
½ cup water
¼ cup sugar
2 tbsp. fresh lemon juice
1 tbsp. butter
2 cups plain 2% reduced-fat Greek yogurt

Combine berries, water, sugar and juice in a small saucepan. Bring mixture to a boil. Reduce heat to medium-low; gently boil 10 minutes or until sauce thickens. Stir in butter. Spoon ½ cup yogurt into each of 4 bowls; top each serving with about ¼ cup sauce. Serve immediately. Serves 4. (*Note*: This is also a wonderful dessert.)

Nutritional Information: 192 calories; 5.8g fat; 11.8g protein; 25.7g carbohydrate; 2g dietary fiber; 14.3mg cholesterol; 64mg sodium.

Lunch

Creamy Chicken Salad

⅔ cup plain 2% reduced-fat Greek yogurt
¼ cup red onion, finely chopped
1 tbsp. fresh lemon juice

2 tsp. fresh dill, chopped
½ tsp. salt
½ tsp. black pepper, freshly ground
1 cucumber, seeded and shredded
1 garlic clove, minced
2 cups rotisserie chicken breast, shredded, skinless and boneless
3 oz. multigrain pita chips

Combine all ingredients but chicken and pita chips in medium bowl, stirring with a whisk. Add chicken; toss to coat. Serve with pita chips. Serves 4.

Nutritional Information: 230 calories; 7.5g fat; 23g protein; 18.7g carbohydrate; 2.1g dietary fiber; 53mg cholesterol; 569mg sodium.

Dinner

Beefsteak with Mustard Sauce
1 lb. flank steak, trimmed
½ tsp. salt
½ tsp. black pepper, freshly ground
1 tsp. canola oil
1½ tsp. fresh garlic cloves, minced
2 tbsp. lower-sodium soy sauce
1 tsp. Dijon mustard
¾ tsp. sugar
1½ tbsp. heavy whipping cream
2 tbsp. fresh cilantro, chopped and divided
nonstick cooking spray

Heat a grill pan over high heat. Sprinkle steak evenly with salt and pepper. Lightly coat steak with nonstick cooking spray. Add steak to pan; grill for 5 minutes on each side or until desired degree of doneness. Let stand 3 minutes. Heat a small skillet over medium-high heat. Add oil to pan; swirl to coat. Add garlic; cook for 30 seconds or until fragrant. Add soy sauce, mustard and sugar; cook 1 minute or until bubbly. Remove pan from heat. Stir in cream and 1 tablespoon cilantro. Cut steak diagonally across grain into thin slices. Sprinkle with remaining 1 tablespoon cilantro. Serve sauce with steak. Serves 4.

Nutritional Information: 202 calories; 9.7g fat; 25g protein; 2.3g carbohydrate; 0.1g dietary fiber; 45mg cholesterol; 541mg sodium.

Garlic Mashed Potatoes
2 lbs. red potatoes, cubed and peeled
2 garlic cloves, halved
½ cup nonfat milk
1 tbsp. butter
¼ tsp. salt
¼ tsp. black pepper

Place potatoes and garlic in a medium saucepan; cover with cold water. Bring to a boil. Reduce heat and simmer 12 minutes or until potatoes are very tender. Drain. Return potato mixture to pan. Add milk, 1 tablespoon butter, salt and black pepper; mash with a potato masher to desired consistency. Serves 4.

Nutritional Information: 195 calories; 2.8g fat; 5.4g protein; 38.1g carbohydrate; 3.9g dietary fiber; 10mg cholesterol; 194mg sodium.

DAY 5

Breakfast
1 cup puffed rice cereal
1 cup nonfat milk
½ cup strawberries, sliced
1 cup orange juice

Nutritional Information: 276 calories; 1g fat; 11g protein; 56g carbohydrate; 3g dietary fiber; 4mg cholesterol; 130mg sodium.

Lunch

Green Bean Salad with Rotisserie Chicken
4 oz. French bread baguette, cut into 12 thin slices
1½ cups green beans, trimmed and cut in half
3 tbsp. extra-virgin olive oil
1½ tbsp. fresh lemon juice
1½ tbsp. Dijon mustard
1 tsp. fresh thyme, chopped
¼ tsp. salt
½ tsp. black pepper, freshly ground
2 cups rotisserie chicken (white and dark meat), shredded, skinless and boneless
1 cup cherry tomatoes, halved

Preheat broiler. Arrange bread in a single layer on a baking sheet. Broil 1 minute or until toasted. Steam green beans 3 minutes or until crisp-tender. Drain. Rinse with cold water; drain. Combine oil, lemon juice, mustard, thyme, salt and pepper in a medium bowl; stir with a whisk. Add chicken, beans and tomatoes; toss to combine. Serve with toast. Serves 4.

Nutritional Information: 286 calories; 14.3g fat; 18.4g protein; 22.6g carbohydrate; 2.5g dietary fiber; 62mg cholesterol; 633mg sodium.

Dinner

Broccoli Bacon Mac and Cheese
3 cups broccoli florets
8 oz. rigatoni, uncooked
1 tbsp. butter
1½ tbsp. all-purpose flour
1¼ cups nonfat milk
¼ cup green onions, thinly sliced
2 oz. processed American cheese, light, cut into pieces

½ tsp. salt
2 slices center-cut bacon, cooked and crumbled
¼ tsp. black pepper, freshly ground
2 oz. cheddar cheese, shredded (about ½ cup packed)

Steam broccoli 5 minutes or until crisp-tender; drain. Pat dry and keep warm. Cook pasta in boiling water in a large saucepan for 8 minutes or until *al dente*; drain and keep warm. Wipe pan with paper towels and return to medium heat. Melt butter in pan. Sprinkle flour over melted butter; cook for 1 minute, stirring constantly with a whisk. Gradually add milk to the flour mixture in pan and bring to a boil, stirring constantly with a whisk. Cook for 1 minute or until slightly thick and remove from heat. Add American cheese; stir until smooth. Stir in sliced green onions, salt, pepper, cooked bacon and cheddar cheese. Stir in broccoli and pasta. Serve immediately. Serves 4.

Nutritional Information: 403 calories; 11.3g fat; 19.6g protein; 53.4g carbohydrate; 3.8g dietary fiber; 39mg cholesterol; 772mg sodium.

DAY 6

Breakfast
1 (2-oz.) English muffin
1 tsp. margarine, light
1 cup cantaloupe
1 cup nonfat milk

Nutritional Information: 292 calories; 4g fat; 14g protein; 51g carbohydrate; 3g dietary fiber; 4mg cholesterol; 451mg sodium.

Lunch

Shrimp Tacos with Apple Salsa
1½ tbsp. extra-virgin olive oil
4 tsp. fresh lime juice, divided
¼ tsp. cumin, ground
¼ tsp. paprika
1 lb. medium shrimp, peeled and deveined
¼ tsp. red pepper, crushed
⅓ cup green onions, sliced
¼ tsp. salt, divided
½ tsp. lime rind, grated
1 Granny Smith apple, thinly sliced
1 jalapeno pepper, minced and seeded
8 (6-inch) corn tortillas
1 oz. queso fresco, crumbled

Combine 1 tablespoon olive oil, 2 teaspoons lime juice, cumin, paprika and red pepper in a small bowl. Pour into a ziplock bag and add shrimp. Seal bag and mix well. Let stand 15 minutes. For apple salsa, combine 1½ teaspoons oil, 2 teaspoons juice, onions, ⅛ teaspoon salt, lime rind, apple and jalapeño; toss. Set aside. Remove shrimp from bag; discard marinade. Heat a grill pan over medium-high heat. Sprinkle shrimp with ⅛ teaspoon salt. Arrange half of shrimp in pan; grill 2 minutes on each side or until done. Remove from pan; keep warm. Repeat procedure with remaining shrimp. Toast the tortillas in grill pan, if desired. Place 2 tortillas on each of 4 plates and divide shrimp evenly among tortillas. Divide salsa evenly among tacos and top with queso fresco. Serves 4 (2 tacos each).

Nutritional Information: 259 calories; 9.4g fat; 21.2g protein; 24.3g carbohydrate; 3g dietary fiber; 170mg cholesterol; 364mg sodium.

Dinner
Pork Chipotle
½ cup chopped onion
1½ tbsp. honey
1 tsp. cumin, ground
⅛ tsp. cinnamon, ground
9 large garlic cloves, peeled
3 chipotle chiles, canned in adobo sauce
1 lime
2 tbsp. extra-virgin olive oil, divided
1 (1¼-lb.) pork shoulder (Boston butt), boneless and trimmed
¾ tsp. salt
½ cup fat-free chicken broth

In a food processor, combine onion, honey, cumin, cinnamon, garlic and chiles. Pulse until finely chopped. Peel and section lime over a bowl, catching juices; discard peel. Add lime juice, lime sections and 1 tablespoon olive oil to food processor; process until smooth. Scrape the chipotle mixture into a zip-top plastic bag. Add pork; seal. Marinate in refrigerator 1 hour. Preheat oven to 325° F. Heat a small Dutch oven over medium-high heat. Add 1 tablespoon oil to pan; swirl. Remove pork from bag; reserve marinade. Sprinkle pork with salt. Add pork to pan; sauté 8 minutes, browning on all sides. Remove pork from pan. Add broth and reserved marinade to pan; bring to a boil, scraping pan to loosen browned bits. Return pork to pan; cover and bake at 325° F for 2½ hours or until pork is fork-tender. Shred pork; toss with sauce. Serves 4.

Nutritional Information: 344 calories; 22.1g fat; 22.3g protein; 14.1g carbohydrate; 2.3g dietary fiber; 83mg cholesterol; 591mg sodium.

DAY 7

Breakfast
Orange and Banana Smoothie
1 cup orange juice
1 cup vanilla lowfat yogurt
⅛ tsp. cinnamon, ground
1 ripe banana, sliced

Place all ingredients in a blender; process until smooth. Serves 2. (*Note*: A frozen banana makes for a thicker smoothie.)

Nutritional Information: 206 calories; 2g fat; 7.2g protein; 42.1g carbohydrate; 1.7g dietary fiber; 6mg cholesterol; 150mg sodium.

Lunch

Tex-Mex Taco Salad

1 (8.8-oz.) pouch precooked brown rice (such as Uncle Ben's®)
8 oz. ground sirloin
¼ cup water
1½ tbsp. taco seasoning
½ cup corn, whole-kernel, frozen
1 cup tomatoes, chopped
1 (15-oz.) can black beans, organic, rinsed and drained
½ cup onion, chopped
1 jalapeño pepper, minced
4 tsp. fresh cilantro, chopped
6 cups salad greens, mixed

Heat rice according to directions and set aside. Heat a large skillet over medium-high heat. Add beef; cook 3 minutes or until done, stirring to crumble. Stir in ¼ cup water and taco seasoning; bring to a simmer. Stir in corn and beans; cook 1 minute or until heated. Stir in rice. In small bowl, combine tomatoes, onion, pepper and cilantro. Divide salad greens on 4 plates. Top with ¼ meat mixture and ¼ tomato mixture. Serve immediately. Serves 4.

Nutritional Information: 306 calories; 7.6g fat; 18g protein; 44.4g carbohydrate; 4.37g dietary fiber; 37mg cholesterol; 503mg sodium.

Dinner

Pecan-crusted Trout Fillets

2 tbsp. all-purpose flour
¼ cup nonfat buttermilk
⅓ cup pecan halves, ground
⅓ cup panko
4 (6-oz.) trout fillets, divided
½ tsp. salt
½ tsp. black pepper
1 tbsp. butter, divided
1 tbsp. extra-virgin olive oil, divided
1 tbsp. fresh parsley, chopped
4 lemon wedges

Place flour in a shallow dish. Place buttermilk in a dish. Combine pecans and panko in a dish. Sprinkle fish with salt and pepper. Dredge flesh side of 2 fillets in flour; dip in buttermilk. Dredge in panko mixture. Melt 1½ teaspoons butter in a large nonstick skillet over medium-high heat. Add 1½ teaspoons oil. Add dredged fillets, crust-side down; cook 3 minutes on each side or until done. Remove from pan. Repeat procedure with remaining flour, buttermilk, panko mixture, fillets, butter and oil. Top with parsley. Serve with lemon wedges. Serves 4.

Nutritional Information: 355 calories; 20g fat; 32.7g protein; 10.8g carbohydrate; 1.3g dietary fiber; 106mg cholesterol; 439mg sodium.

Creamy Spinach and Mushrooms

4 tsp. canola oil, divided
8 oz. sliced cremini mushrooms
1 (10-oz.) package fresh baby spinach
1/3 cup shallots, finely chopped
2 tsp. fresh garlic, minced
3/4 cup nonfat milk

1 tbsp. all-purpose flour
3/8 tsp. salt
1/4 tsp. black pepper
dash of nutmeg
2½ oz. 1/3-less-fat cream cheese

Heat a large skillet over medium-high heat. Add 1½ teaspoons oil; swirl to coat. Add mushrooms; cook 6 minutes or until liquid evaporates. Remove mushrooms from pan. Add 1½ teaspoons oil to pan; swirl to coat. Add spinach; cook 1 minute or until spinach wilts. Remove from heat. Heat a Dutch oven over medium heat. Add remaining 1 teaspoon oil; swirl to coat. Add shallots and garlic; cook 1 minute, stirring constantly. Combine milk and flour; stir with a whisk. Add milk mixture, salt, pepper and nutmeg to pan. Bring to a boil, stirring constantly. Cook 3 minutes or until thickened, stirring constantly. Add cheese; stir until cheese melts and the mixture is smooth. Add mushrooms and spinach to milk mixture and toss gently to coat. Serve immediately. Serves 4.

Nutritional Information: 102 calories; 6g fat; 4.8g protein; 8.1g carbohydrate; 1.4g dietary fiber; 9mg cholesterol; 241mg sodium.

Second Week Grocery List

Produce
- asparagus
- baby arugula
- baby spinach
- bananas
- basil leaves
- blackberries
- carrots
- celery
- cilantro
- cremini mushrooms
- eggplant
- garlic
- grape tomatoes
- green beans
- green bell peppers
- green onions
- lemons
- mushrooms
- onions
- oregano
- parsley
- portobello mushroom caps
- red bell peppers
- red onion
- shallots
- thyme
- tomatoes
- yellow onion
- Yukon gold or small baking potatoes

Baking/Cooking Products
- baking powder
- canola oil
- dark brown sugar
- flour, all-purpose
- nonstick cooking spray
- olive oil, extra-virgin
- powdered sugar
- sugar
- vanilla extract

Spices
- basil
- black pepper
- chili powder
- coriander
- cumin
- mustard, dry
- garlic powder
- Italian seasoning
- onion powder
- oregano
- paprika
- red pepper
- salt
- turmeric

Nuts/Seeds
- hazelnuts
- pine nuts
- walnuts

Condiments, Spreads and Sauces
- barbecue sauce
- Dijon mustard
- honey
- hummus, plain or flavored
- ketchup
- maple syrup
- marinara sauce, lower-sodium
- mustard
- peanut butter, creamy
- sherry vinegar
- soy sauce, lower-sodium

- [ ] strawberry jam
- [ ] white wine vinegar
- [ ] Worcestershire sauce

Breads, Cereals and Pasta
- [ ] bagel
- [ ] brown rice (such as Uncle Ben's®)
- [ ] elbow macaroni
- [ ] fettuccine
- [ ] French bread, whole-wheat
- [ ] Grape Nuts® cereal
- [ ] hoagie rolls
- [ ] panko (Japanese breadcrumbs)
- [ ] pizza dough, fresh
- [ ] slider buns
- [ ] sourdough bread
- [ ] tortillas, corn
- [ ] wheat flakes cereal
- [ ] white bread
- [ ] white rice, long-grain

Canned/Frozen Foods
- [ ] asparagus spears
- [ ] beef broth, fat-free, lower-sodium
- [ ] crushed tomatoes
- [ ] exotic mushroom blend (such as shiitake, cremini and oyster)
- [ ] green peas
- [ ] jalapeño pepper
- [ ] kalamata olives
- [ ] peaches
- [ ] potato wedges
- [ ] refried beans, fat-free
- [ ] tomatoes and green chilies, mild and diced

Dairy Products
- [ ] Asiago cheese
- [ ] butter
- [ ] buttermilk, nonfat
- [ ] cheddar jack cheese, reduced-fat
- [ ] cottage cheese, nonfat
- [ ] cream cheese, 1/3-less-fat
- [ ] goat cheese
- [ ] Greek yogurt, 2% reduced-fat, plain
- [ ] half-and-half
- [ ] Manchego cheese
- [ ] milk, nonfat
- [ ] Monterey Jack cheese with jalapeño peppers
- [ ] mozzarella cheese, part-skim
- [ ] Parmigiano-Reggiano cheese
- [ ] provolone cheese
- [ ] ricotta cheese, part-skim
- [ ] ricotta cheese, whole-milk
- [ ] sharp cheddar cheese
- [ ] sour cream, reduced-fat
- [ ] yogurt, plain, fat-free

Juices
- [ ] apple juice
- [ ] lemon juice
- [ ] lime juice

Meat and Poultry
- [ ] crawfish meat, cooked and frozen
- [ ] egg substitute
- [ ] egg white
- [ ] eggs
- [ ] flank steak
- [ ] ground round
- [ ] ground sirloin
- [ ] halibut fillets
- [ ] hot dogs, turkey
- [ ] Italian sausage, turkey
- [ ] pork, lean-ground
- [ ] prosciutto, thin slices
- [ ] rotisserie chicken breast
- [ ] shrimp

Second Week Meals and Recipes

DAY 1

Breakfast

Blackberry Smoothie

2 cups fresh or frozen blackberries
1 cup plain fat-free yogurt
1 cup apple juice
¼ cup honey
1 large ripe banana

Combine all ingredients in a blender; process until smooth. Strain blackberry mixture through a sieve; discard seeds. Serves 3.

Nutritional Information: 265 calories; 0.8g fat; 5.7g protein; 63.2g carbohydrate; 8.7g dietary fiber; 2mg cholesterol; 62mg sodium.

Lunch

Cheesesteak Hoagie

1 (12-oz.) flank steak, trimmed
¼ tsp. salt
½ tsp. black pepper, freshly ground
2 (5-inch) portobello mushroom caps
2 tsp. extra-virgin olive oil, divided
1 cup onion, thinly sliced
1½ cups green bell pepper, thinly sliced
2 tsp. garlic, minced
½ tsp. Worcestershire sauce
½ tsp. lower-sodium soy sauce
2 tsp. all-purpose flour
½ cup nonfat milk
1 oz. provolone cheese, torn into small pieces
2 tbsp. Parmigiano-Reggiano cheese, grated
¼ tsp. dry mustard
4 (3-oz.) hoagie rolls, toasted

Place beef in freezer for 15 minutes. Cut beef across the grain into thin slices. Sprinkle beef with salt and pepper. Remove brown gills from the undersides of mushroom caps using a spoon; discard gills. Remove stems; discard. Thinly slice mushroom caps; cut slices in half crosswise. Heat a large nonstick skillet over medium-high heat. Add 1 teaspoon oil to pan; swirl to coat. Add beef to pan; sauté 2 minutes or until beef loses its pink color, stirring constantly. Remove beef from pan. Add remaining 1 teaspoon oil to pan. Add onion; sauté 3 minutes. Add mushrooms, bell pepper and garlic; sauté 6 minutes. Return beef to pan; sauté 1 minute or until thoroughly heated and vegetables are tender. Remove from heat. Stir in Worcestershire and soy sauce; keep warm. Place flour in a small saucepan; gradually add milk, stirring with a whisk until blended. Bring to a simmer over medium heat; cook 1 minute or until slightly thickened. Remove from heat. Add cheeses and mustard, stirring until smooth. Keep warm (mixture will thicken as it cools). Hollow out top and bottom halves of bread, leaving a ½-inch-thick shell; reserve torn bread for another use. Divide the beef mixture evenly among bottom halves of hoagies. Drizzle sauce evenly over beef mixture; replace top halves. Serves 4.

Nutritional Information: 397 calories; 12.4g fat; 30.8g protein; 44.1g carbohydrate; 3.7g dietary fiber; 37mg cholesterol; 637mg sodium.

Dinner

Ricotta and Spinach Pasta

9 oz. fettuccine, refrigerated
⅔ cup whole-milk ricotta cheese
1 tsp. lemon rind, grated
¾ tsp. salt, divided
½ tsp. black pepper
½ tsp. red pepper, crushed
2 tbsp. extra-virgin olive oil, divided

1½ cups red bell pepper, diced
1 cup mushrooms, sliced
⅓ cup walnuts, chopped
4 garlic cloves, thinly sliced
1 tbsp. fresh lemon juice
3 cups fresh baby spinach
lemon rind strips (optional)

Cook pasta according to package directions. Drain in a colander over a bowl; reserve ½ cup pasta water. In small bowl, combine ricotta, lemon rind, ¼ teaspoon salt and red and black pepper. Heat 1 tablespoon oil in a large skillet over medium-high heat. Add bell pepper and mushrooms; sauté 2 minutes. Add walnuts, ½ teaspoon salt and garlic; sauté 2 minutes. Stir in 1 tablespoon oil and juice. Add pasta, pasta water and spinach; cook 1 minute or until spinach wilts. Top with ricotta mixture and rind strips, if desired. Serves 4.

Nutritional Information: 412 calories; 20.5g fat; 15g protein; 43.2g carbohydrate; 4.3g dietary fiber; 59mg cholesterol; 442mg sodium.

DAY 2

Breakfast

Peanut Butter and Jelly Muffins

1 cup all-purpose flour
¾ cup all-purpose flour

¼ cup sugar
¼ cup dark brown sugar, packed

1 tbsp. baking powder
½ tsp. salt
1¼ cups nonfat milk
⅓ cup creamy peanut butter
¼ cup egg substitute

2 tbsp. butter, melted
1 tsp. vanilla extract
¼ cup strawberry jam
nonstick cooking spray

Preheat oven to 400° F. Lightly spoon flours into dry measuring cups; level with a knife. Combine flours, sugars, baking powder and salt in a large bowl; stir with a whisk. Make a well in the center of the mixture. Combine milk, peanut butter, egg substitute, butter and vanilla extract; add to flour mixture, stirring just until moist. Spoon batter into 12 muffin cups coated with nonstick cooking spray. Fill each cup half full with batter. Spoon 1 teaspoon jam into each cup. Spoon remaining batter on top to cover jam. Bake at 400° F for 20 minutes or until muffins spring back when touched lightly in center. Let cool in pan 5 minutes. Remove from pan and cool on a wire rack. Serves 12.

Nutritional Information: 185 calories; 5.8g fat; 5.2g protein; 29.4g carbohydrate; 1.6g dietary fiber; 5.6mg cholesterol; 288mg sodium.

Lunch

Mushroom Cheese Panini

1 tsp. butter
¼ cup shallots, minced
1 tbsp. fresh thyme, chopped
2 tsp. fresh garlic, minced
½ tsp. black pepper, freshly ground
¼ tsp. salt
1 (8-oz.) package pre-sliced cremini mushrooms

2 (4-oz.) packages pre-sliced exotic mushroom blend (such as shiitake, cremini and oyster)
1½ tbsp. sherry vinegar
8 (1½-oz.) slices sourdough bread
3 oz. Manchego cheese, shaved
1 garlic clove, halved
nonstick cooking spray

Melt butter in a large skillet over medium-high heat; add shallots, thyme, garlic, pepper, salt and mushrooms. Cook 10 minutes or until mushrooms are tender and liquid almost evaporates, stirring frequently. Add vinegar; cook 30 seconds or until liquid almost evaporates. Divide the mushroom mixture evenly among four bread slices. Top evenly with Manchego cheese and remaining bread slices. Heat a large grill pan over medium-high heat. Coat pan with nonstick cooking spray. Add sandwiches to pan. Place a cast-iron or heavy skillet on top of sandwiches; press gently to flatten. Cook sandwiches 2 minutes on each side or until cheese melts and bread is toasted (leave the skillet on the sandwiches while they cook). Rub the top and bottom of each sandwich with cut side of garlic clove. Serves 4.

Nutritional Information: 352 calories; 11g fat; 16.8g protein; 48.8g carbohydrate; 3.7g dietary fiber; 25mg cholesterol; 741mg sodium.

Dinner

Meatloaf Surprise

1½ oz. whole-wheat French bread, torn into pieces
½ cup ketchup, divided
1 cup onion, coarsely chopped
5 tbsp. fresh flat-leaf parsley, chopped and divided
¼ cup nonfat buttermilk
1 tbsp. Dijon mustard
1 tbsp. garlic (about 3 cloves), minced
½ tsp. black pepper, freshly ground
¼ tsp. salt
2 oz. sharp cheddar cheese, diced
2 large eggs, lightly beaten
1 lb. ground sirloin
nonstick cooking spray

Preheat oven to 350° F. Place bread in a food processor; pulse 10 times or until coarse crumbs measure 1 cup. Arrange breadcrumbs in an even layer on a baking sheet. Bake at 350° F for 6 minutes or until lightly toasted; cool. Combine toasted breadcrumbs, ¼ cup ketchup, onion, 3 tablespoons parsley, buttermilk, garlic, Dijon mustard, black pepper, salt, cheddar cheese, eggs and sirloin in a bowl; gently mix until just combined. Transfer the mixture to a 9" x 5" loaf pan coated with nonstick cooking spray; do not pack. Bake at 350° F for 30 minutes. Brush top of loaf with remaining ¼ cup ketchup. Bake an additional 25 minutes or until thermometer registers 160° F. Let stand for 10 minutes and cut into 6 slices. Sprinkle with remaining parsley. Serves 6.

Nutritional Information: 258 calories; 12.6g fat; 21.2g protein; 14g carbohydrate; 0.8g dietary fiber; 119mg cholesterol; 557mg sodium.

Green Beans with Toasted Garlic

1 lb. green beans, trimmed
2 tsp. butter
1 tsp. extra-virgin olive oil
4 garlic cloves, thinly sliced
¼ tsp. salt
½ tsp. black pepper

Bring a large saucepan of water to a boil. Add beans; cook 5 minutes. Plunge beans into ice water; drain. Heat a large skillet over medium-high heat. Add butter and oil; swirl until butter melts. Add garlic; sauté 30 seconds. Remove garlic; set aside. Add beans; sprinkle with salt and pepper. Cook 2 minutes, tossing frequently. Top with garlic. Serves 4.

Nutritional Information: 67 calories; 3.2g fat; 2.3g protein; 9.2g carbohydrate; 4g dietary fiber; 5mg cholesterol; 169mg sodium.

DAY 3

Breakfast

1 cup wheat flakes cereal
1 cup nonfat milk
½ medium banana, sliced

Nutritional Information: 265 calories; 3g fat; 18g protein; 63g carbohydrate; 26g dietary fiber; 4mg cholesterol; 128mg sodium.

Lunch

Meatball Sliders

1 tbsp. extra-virgin olive oil, divided
3 garlic cloves, minced
3 shallots, finely diced
⅓ cup part-skim ricotta cheese
¼ cup fresh parsley, chopped
¼ cup panko, toasted
½ tsp. black pepper, freshly ground
¼ tsp. red pepper, crushed
⅛ tsp. salt
8 oz. lean-ground pork
2 (4-oz.) links turkey Italian sausage, with casings removed
1 large egg
1½ cups lower-sodium marinara sauce
12 slider buns, toasted
12 basil leaves

Heat 1 teaspoon oil in a large skillet over medium heat; swirl to coat. Add garlic and shallots to pan; sauté 3 minutes or until shallots are softened, stirring frequently. Combine shallot mixture, ricotta, parsley, breadcrumbs, peppers, salt, ground pork, sausage and egg in a medium bowl. Shape mixture into 12 (1-inch) meatballs; flatten each meatball slightly. Return pan to medium-high heat. Add remaining 2 teaspoons oil to pan. Add meatballs to pan; cook 6 minutes, turning once. Add marinara sauce; bring to a boil, scraping pan to loosen browned bits. Cover, reduce heat and simmer 8 minutes or until meatballs are done. Top bottom half of each bun with 1½ tablespoons sauce, 1 meatball, 1 basil leaf and top half of bun. Serves 6.

Nutritional Information: 429 calories; 16.3g fat; 25.4g protein; 60.5g carbohydrate; 2.3g dietary fiber; 85mg cholesterol; 764mg sodium.

Dinner

Shrimp with Peas and Rice

1 (8.8-oz.) pouch precooked brown rice (such as Uncle Ben's®)
1 tbsp. extra-virgin olive oil
8 oz. medium shrimp, peeled and deveined
3 garlic cloves, minced

¼ cup water
⅔ cup green peas, frozen
1 tbsp. white wine vinegar
¾ tsp. salt

¼ tsp. red pepper, crushed
¼ tsp. turmeric, ground
2 tbsp. fresh flat-leaf parsley, chopped

Heat rice according to directions; set aside. Heat oil in a large skillet over medium-high heat. Add shrimp; sauté 2 minutes. Add garlic; sauté 1 minute or until shrimp are done. Remove mixture from pan. Bring water to a simmer. Add peas; cover and cook 2 minutes or until done. Stir in rice, shrimp, vinegar, salt, pepper and turmeric; cook 1 minute or until heated. Sprinkle with parsley. Serves 3.

Nutritional Information: 280 calories; 8.4g fat; 20.2g protein; 30.5g carbohydrate; 2.8g dietary fiber; 115mg cholesterol; 629mg sodium.

Roasted Carrots

2 cups carrots, (2-inch) diagonally cut
1 tbsp. butter, melted
1 tsp. extra-virgin olive oil

¼ tsp. salt
¼ tsp. black pepper
nonstick cooking spray

Preheat oven to 425° F. Combine all ingredients on a baking sheet coated with nonstick cooking spray. Toss gently to coat. Bake for 15 minutes or until tender. Serves 4.

Nutritional Information: 61 calories; 4.2g fat; 0.6g protein; 5.9g carbohydrate; 1.7g dietary fiber; 8mg cholesterol; 183mg sodium.

DAY 4

Breakfast

½ bagel, toasted
1 tbsp. creamy peanut butter

½ medium banana, sliced
1 cup nonfat milk

Nutritional Information: 358 calories; 10g fat; 18g protein; 53g carbohydrate; 3g dietary fiber; 4mg cholesterol; 440mg sodium.

Lunch

Chicken and Asiago Salad

2 (1-oz.) slices sourdough bread, cut into ½-inch cubes

½ tsp. dried basil
⅛ tsp. garlic powder

3 tbsp. extra-virgin olive oil, divided
2 oz. prosciutto, thin slices and chopped
2 tbsp. lemon juice
¼ tsp. salt
2 (5-oz.) packages baby arugula
1½ oz. Asiago cheese, shaved and divided (about ⅓ cup)
6 oz. rotisserie chicken breast, shredded, skinless and boneless
1 cup grape tomatoes, halved
nonstick cooking spray

Preheat oven to 425° F. Place bread cubes on a baking sheet and lightly coat with nonstick cooking spray. Add basil and garlic powder; toss well. Place bread mixture in preheated oven; bake for 8 minutes or until crisp. Heat a large nonstick skillet over medium-high heat. Add 1 teaspoon oil to pan; swirl to coat. Add prosciutto; sauté 4 minutes or until prosciutto is crisp. Drain on paper towels. Combine remaining 2 tablespoons plus 2 teaspoons oil, juice and salt in a small bowl; stir well with a whisk. Place arugula, half of cheese and juice mixture in a large bowl; toss well to coat. Divide arugula mixture evenly among 6 plates; divide chicken, prosciutto, tomatoes, remaining cheese and croutons evenly over salads. Serves 6.

Nutritional Information: 193 calories; 11.5g fat; 14.4g protein; 8.9g carbohydrate; 1.5g dietary fiber; 37mg cholesterol; 481mg sodium.

Dinner

Tex Mac and Cheese

1 tsp. canola oil
¾ lb. ground round
1 tsp. garlic powder
1 tsp. coriander, ground
1 tsp. cumin, ground
2 tsp. chili powder
2 cups fat-free, lower-sodium beef broth
1 cup water
1 (10-oz.) can mild tomatoes and green chiles, undrained and diced
8 oz. uncooked elbow macaroni
½ cup nonfat milk
4 oz. ⅓-less-fat cream cheese
4½ oz. reduced-fat cheddar jack cheese, finely shredded

Heat a Dutch oven over medium-high heat. Add oil. Add beef, garlic powder, cumin, coriander and chili powder; cook 3 minutes. Add broth, water and tomatoes; bring to a boil. Stir in macaroni; cover and cook 10 minutes or until macaroni is done. Heat milk and cream cheese in a saucepan over medium heat. Cook 4 minutes or until cheese melts, stirring frequently. Remove from heat. Stir in cheddar. Add cheese sauce to macaroni mixture; toss well to coat. Serves 6.

Nutritional Information: 342 calories; 12.3g fat; 25.7g protein; 32.7g carbohydrate; 1.8g dietary fiber; 60mg cholesterol; 652mg sodium.

DAY 5

Breakfast

Breakfast Tacos with Homemade Salsa

1 cup tomato, chopped
¼ cup red onion, chopped
2 tbsp. fresh cilantro, chopped
1 tsp. jalapeño pepper, minced
¼ tsp. salt
4 tsp. lime juice, divided
1 tsp. garlic, minced and divided
1 cup fat-free refried beans
¼ tsp. cumin, ground
1 tbsp. nonfat milk
6 large eggs, lightly beaten
¼ cup green onions, chopped
8 (6-inch) corn tortillas
½ cup (2 oz.) Monterey Jack cheese with jalapeño peppers, shredded
8 tsp. reduced-fat sour cream
nonstick cooking spray

For salsa, combine tomato, onion, cilantro, jalapeno and salt. Stir in 2 teaspoons lime juice and ½ teaspoon garlic. In another bowl, combine beans, remaining 2 teaspoons juice, remaining ½ teaspoon garlic and cumin. Combine milk and eggs in a medium bowl; stir with a whisk. Heat a large nonstick skillet over medium-high heat. Coat pan with nonstick cooking spray. Add green onions to pan; sauté 1 minute, stirring frequently. Stir in egg mixture; cook 3 minutes or until soft-scrambled, stirring constantly. Remove from heat. Warm tortillas according to package directions. Spread 1 tablespoon bean mixture on each tortilla. Spoon about 2 tablespoons egg mixture down the center of each tortilla. Top each serving with 1 tablespoon tomato mixture, 1 tablespoon cheese and 1 teaspoon sour cream. Serves 4 (2 tacos each).

Nutritional Information: 314 calories; 13g fat; 19g protein; 34g carbohydrate; 6.5g dietary fiber; 289mg cholesterol; 407mg sodium.

Lunch

Open-faced Hummus Sandwich

4 (1½-oz.) slices sourdough bread
1½ cups grape tomatoes, quartered
⅓ cup green onions, chopped
1 tbsp. extra-virgin olive oil
¼ cup kalamata olives, pitted and chopped
¼ tsp. black pepper
⅛ tsp. salt

1 garlic clove, minced
½ cup goat cheese, crumbled

1 (8-oz.) container plain or flavored hummus

Preheat broiler. Arrange bread on a baking sheet. Broil 1 minute or until toasted. Combine tomatoes, green onions, olives, olive oil, pepper, salt and garlic. Spread about ¼ cup hummus over each bread slice. Divide tomato mixture evenly among servings. Top each serving with 2 tablespoons cheese. Serves 4.

Nutritional Information: 358 calories; 20g fat; 12.3g protein; 36.5g carbohydrate; 4.3g dietary fiber; 7mg cholesterol; 811mg sodium.

Dinner

Hazelnut Crusted Halibut with Asparagus

1 tbsp. butter
2 tsp. extra-virgin olive oil, divided
4 (6-oz.) halibut fillets, skinned
1 egg white, lightly beaten
½ tsp. salt, divided
½ tsp. black pepper, freshly ground and divided

½ cup hazelnuts, finely chopped
2 garlic cloves, thinly sliced
1 lb. asparagus, trimmed
1 tsp. fresh thyme, chopped
4 lemon wedges
nonstick cooking spray

Preheat oven to 400° F. Heat butter and 1 teaspoon oil in a large nonstick skillet over medium-high heat. Brush tops of fish fillets with egg white; sprinkle fish evenly with ¼ teaspoon salt and ¼ teaspoon pepper. Coat tops of fish with nuts, pressing gently to adhere. Place half of fish, nut side down, in pan; cook 3 minutes or until browned. Turn fish over; cook 4 minutes or until desired degree of doneness. Combine remaining 1 teaspoon olive oil, garlic and asparagus on a jellyroll pan coated with nonstick cooking spray; toss to combine. Sprinkle with remaining ¼ teaspoon salt, remaining ¼ teaspoon pepper and thyme. Bake at 400° F for 8 minutes or until crisp-tender. Serve with fish and lemon wedges. Serves 4.

Nutritional Information: 356 calories; 18g fat; 41.2g protein; 8.2g carbohydrate; 4g dietary fiber; 62mg cholesterol; 424mg sodium.

Roasted Red Potatoes

1 tbsp. extra-virgin olive oil
¼ tsp. salt

½ tsp. black pepper
2 shallots, thinly sliced

1 (20-oz.) bag refrigerated potato wedges or fresh-cut into wedges (with skins)

Preheat oven to 400° F. Combine all ingredients on a large jellyroll pan; toss well. Roast at 400° F for 15 minutes. Toss and cook another 10 to 15 minutes or until fork tender. Serves 4.

Nutritional Information: 123 calories; 3.4g fat; 3.8g protein; 18.8g carbohydrate; 3.5g dietary fiber; 0.0mg cholesterol; 269mg sodium.

DAY 6

Breakfast

1 cup peach slices in light syrup, drained
1 cup nonfat cottage cheese
¼ cup Grape Nuts® cereal (sprinkled over yogurt and peaches)

Nutritional Information: 349 calories; trace fat; 34g protein; 58g carbohydrate; 5g dietary fiber; 10mg cholesterol; 806mg sodium.

Lunch

Pigs in a Blanket

1 (6-oz.) portion fresh pizza dough
1½ oz. part-skim mozzarella cheese, shredded
4 turkey hot dogs, halved crosswise
2 tbsp. ketchup
1 tbsp. barbecue sauce
1 tsp. mustard
nonstick cooking spray

Preheat oven to 425° F. Let dough stand, covered, for 20 minutes. On a lightly floured surface, roll the dough into a 12" x 4" rectangle. Cut rectangle into 4 (4" x 3") rectangles; cut each rectangle in half diagonally to form 8 triangles. Divide cheese evenly among triangles; place in the center of wide ends. Place hot dog half at the wide end of each triangle; roll up, pinching ends to seal. Arrange rolls on a baking sheet coated with nonstick cooking spray. Bake at 425° F for 12 minutes. Combine ketchup, barbecue sauce and mustard. Serve with rolls. Serves 4.

Nutritional Information: 215 calories; 6.2g fat; 13.5g protein; 27.5g carbohydrate; 0.8g dietary fiber; 32mg cholesterol; 825mg sodium.

Dinner

Stuffed Bell Peppers

4 medium red bell peppers
1 tsp. black pepper, divided
½ cup fat-free, lower-sodium beef broth, divided
1 cup cooked long-grain white rice, cooled
½ tsp. salt
1 tsp. Italian seasoning
¾ lb. ground sirloin
2 cups water
2 tsp. extra-virgin olive oil
½ cup fresh parsley, chopped and divided
¾ cup onion, chopped
1 tsp. garlic, minced
1 cup canned crushed tomatoes
¼ cup water
¼ tsp. sugar
¼ tsp. dried oregano
⅛ tsp. red pepper, crushed
2 tbsp. plain 2% reduced-fat Greek yogurt

Preheat oven to 400° F. Cut tops off bell peppers; reserve. Discard seeds. Place peppers in a microwave-safe baking dish; cover with damp paper towels. Microwave at high for 6 minutes. Let stand 5 minutes. Combine ½ teaspoon black pepper, ¼ cup broth, rice, salt, Italian seasoning and beef. Divide beef mixture among peppers; top with tops. Pour 2 cups water into dish; cover. Bake at 400° F for 45 minutes. Sprinkle peppers with ¼ cup parsley. While the peppers cook, heat a medium skillet over medium-high heat. Add oil to pan. Add onion and sauté for 8 minutes, stirring occasionally. Add garlic; sauté for 30 seconds. Add ½ teaspoon black pepper, ¼ cup broth, tomatoes, water, sugar, oregano and red pepper; bring to a boil. Reduce heat; simmer 30 minutes. Stir in ¼ cup parsley and yogurt. Spoon on top of cooked peppers and serve. Serves 4.

Nutritional Information: 454 calories; 12g fat; 25.2g protein; 60g carbohydrate; 6.2g dietary fiber; 56mg cholesterol; 507mg sodium.

DAY 7

Breakfast

French Toast Soufflé

10 cups (1-inch) sturdy white bread, cubed (about 16 [1-oz.] slices)
8 large eggs
1 (8-oz.) block ⅓-less-fat-cream cheese, softened
1½ cups nonfat milk

⅔ cup half-and-half
½ cup maple syrup
½ tsp. vanilla extract

2 tbsp. powdered sugar
¾ cup maple syrup
nonstick cooking spray

Place bread cubes in a 13" x 9" baking dish coated with nonstick cooking spray. Beat cream cheese at medium speed of mixer until smooth. Add eggs, 1 at a time, mixing well after each addition. Add milk, half-and-half, ½ cup maple syrup and vanilla; mix until smooth. Pour cream cheese mixture over top of bread; cover and refrigerate overnight. Preheat oven to 375° F. Remove bread mixture from refrigerator; let stand on counter for 30 minutes. Bake at 375° F for 50 minutes or until set. Sprinkle the soufflé with powdered sugar, and serve with maple syrup. Serves 12.

Nutritional Information: 322 calories; 9.2g fat; 11.6g protein; 51.7g carbohydrate; 2.7g dietary fiber; 169mg cholesterol; 396mg sodium.

Lunch

Cajun Stuffed Baked Potatoes

6 medium Yukon gold or small baking potatoes (about 3 lbs.)
2 tbsp. extra-virgin olive oil, divided
1½ cups yellow onion, chopped
¾ cup green bell pepper, chopped
½ cup celery, thinly sliced
1 tbsp. garlic, minced
¾ tsp. salt
¾ tsp. paprika

½ tsp. onion powder
½ tsp. red pepper, crushed
¾ cup (6 oz.) ⅓-less-fat cream cheese, softened
2 tbsp. butter, softened
1 tbsp. fresh oregano, chopped
2 tsp. fresh thyme, chopped
1½ lbs. frozen cooked crawfish meat, thawed (or cooked shrimp)

Preheat oven to 450° F. Pierce potatoes with a fork; brush with 1 teaspoon olive oil. Bake at 450° F for 50 minutes or until tender. Remove potatoes from oven; cool slightly. Cut potatoes in half lengthwise and scoop pulp out of skins, leaving a ¼-inch-thick shell. Place pulp in a large bowl; coarsely mash pulp. Preheat broiler to high. Heat a large skillet over medium-high heat. Add remaining 5 teaspoons oil to pan; swirl to coat. Add onion, bell pepper and celery to pan; sauté for 4 minutes. Add garlic, salt, paprika, onion powder and red pepper; sauté 1 minute. Remove from heat. Add cheese, butter and herbs, stirring until smooth. Stir cheese mixture and crawfish into potato pulp. Place ½ cup crawfish mixture in each potato shell. Arrange stuffed potatoes on a baking sheet. Broil for 5 minutes or until browned. Serves 6.

Nutritional Information: 451 calories; 16.5g fat; 27.8g protein; 46.8g carbohydrate; 2.9g dietary fiber; 182mg cholesterol; 546mg sodium.

Dinner

Eggplant Roll-ups

1 tbsp. extra-virgin olive oil
2 lbs. tomatoes, seeded and coarsely chopped (about 3 large)
½ tsp. salt, divided
4 garlic cloves, crushed and divided
12 (¼-inch thick) slices eggplant, peeled and cut lengthwise (about 2 medium)
½ tsp. black pepper, freshly ground
2 tbsp. pine nuts, lightly toasted
1 oz. whole-wheat French bread, toasted and torn into pieces
8 oz. part-skim ricotta cheese
1 tsp. lemon rind, grated
1 large egg
¾ cup fresh basil leaves, chopped and divided
2 oz. Parmigiano-Reggiano cheese, grated (about ½ cup) and divided
nonstick cooking spray

Combine oil and tomatoes in a medium saucepan; stir in ¼ teaspoon salt and 2 garlic cloves. Bring to a boil over medium-high heat; reduce heat and simmer 15 minutes or until reduced to 2 cups. Cool 10 minutes. Place mixture in a food processor; process until smooth. Set aside. Preheat broiler to high. Sprinkle eggplant slices evenly with ¼ teaspoon salt and pepper; arrange slices in a single layer on a foil-lined baking sheet. Lightly coat eggplant with nonstick cooking spray. Broil 4 minutes on each side or until lightly browned. Cool 10 minutes. Preheat oven to 375° F. Place remaining 2 garlic cloves in a mini food processor; pulse until chopped. Add nuts and bread; pulse 10 times or until coarse crumbs form. Add ricotta, rind and egg; process until smooth. Stir in ½ cup basil and ¼ cup Parmigiano-Reggiano cheese. Spread 1½ cups tomato sauce over the bottom of an 8-inch square glass or ceramic baking dish coated with nonstick cooking spray. Spread 2 tablespoons ricotta mixture onto each eggplant slice; roll up jellyroll fashion. Place rolls, seam sides down, over sauce in dish. Spoon remaining sauce over rolls. Sprinkle with remaining ¼ cup Parmigiano-Reggiano cheese. Bake at 375° F for 25 minutes or until bubbly. Sprinkle with remaining basil. Serves 4 (3 rolls each).

Nutritional Information: 323 calories; 16.2g fat; 18.3g protein; 32.3g carbohydrate; 12.4g dietary fiber; 79mg cholesterol; 442mg sodium.

Garlic Asparagus

1 lb. asparagus spears, trimmed
1 tbsp. extra-virgin olive oil
2 garlic cloves, thinly sliced
⅛ tsp. salt
¼ tsp. black pepper, freshly ground

Steam asparagus 4 minutes or until crisp-tender. While asparagus steams, heat oil in a large skillet over medium heat. Add garlic; cook 2 minutes or until fragrant, stirring frequently. Add asparagus, salt and pepper; toss to combine. Serves 4.

Nutritional Information: 57 calories; 3.4g fat; 2.5g protein; 5.4g carbohydrate; 2.5g dietary fiber; 0.0mg cholesterol; 74mg sodium.

SNACKS & DESSERTS
(Note: You will need to add these items to the grocery lists.)

Tropical Sherbet

1 (12-oz.) package frozen mango chunks (about 2½ cups)
1 cup frozen pineapple chunks
1 (6-oz.) carton lemon low-fat yogurt
1 tsp. lime rind, grated

Remove mango and pineapple from freezer; let stand at room temperature 10 minutes. Combine mango, pineapple, yogurt and rind in a food processor; process until smooth. Serve immediately (for soft-serve texture) or freeze in an airtight container for 1 hour 30 minutes (for firmer texture). Serves 4.

Nutritional Information: 144 calories; 0.6g fat; 3g protein; 34g carbohydrate; 2.5g dietary fiber; 2mg cholesterol; 78mg sodium.

Texas Sheet Cake

2 cups plus 2 tsp. all-purpose flour
2 cups sugar
1 tsp. baking soda
1 tsp. cinnamon, ground
¼ tsp. salt
¾ cup water
½ cup butter
½ cup unsweetened cocoa, divided
½ cup low-fat buttermilk
1 tbsp. vanilla extract, divided
2 large eggs
6 tbsp. butter
⅓ cup nonfat milk
3 cups powdered sugar
¼ cup chopped pecans, toasted
nonstick cooking spray

Preheat oven to 375° F. Coat a 15" x 10" jellyroll pan with nonstick cooking spray; dust with 2 teaspoons flour. Set aside. Weigh or lightly spoon

2 cups flour into dry measuring cups; level with a knife. Combine flour, sugar, soda, cinnamon and salt in a large bowl. Combine ¾ cup water, ½ cup butter and ¼ cup cocoa in a saucepan; bring to a boil, stirring frequently. Pour into flour mixture. Beat with a mixer at medium speed until well blended. Add buttermilk, 1 teaspoon vanilla and eggs; beat well. Pour batter into prepared pan. Bake at 375° F for 17 minutes or until a wooden pick inserted in center comes out clean. Place on a wire rack. For icing, combine 6 tablespoons butter, nonfat milk, and ¼ cup cocoa in a saucepan. Bring to a boil, stirring constantly. Remove from heat. Gradually stir in powdered sugar; stir in 2 teaspoons vanilla and pecans. Spread over hot cake. Cool completely on a wire rack. Serves 20.

Nutritional Information: 298 calories; 10g fat; 3.1g protein; 49.8g carbohydrate; 0.5g dietary fiber; 44mg cholesterol; 188mg sodium.

Oatmeal Snack Cake

½ cup lowfat buttermilk
½ cup steel-cut oats
½ cup oat flour
1 cup all-purpose flour
1 tsp. baking powder
½ tsp. baking soda
½ tsp. salt
⅔ cup brown sugar, packed
¼ cup butter, softened
1½ tsp. vanilla extract
1 large egg
1 tbsp. powdered sugar (optional)
nonstick cooking spray

Combine buttermilk and oats; cover and refrigerate 8 hours. Preheat oven to 375° F. Lightly spoon flours into a dry measuring cup; level with a knife. Combine flours, baking powder, baking soda and salt, stirring with a whisk. Place sugar and butter in a large bowl; beat with a mixer at medium speed until light and fluffy. Add vanilla and egg; beat until well blended. Stir in oat mixture; beat until well blended. Add flour mixture, beating just until moist. Spoon batter into a 13" x 9" baking pan coated with nonstick cooking spray. Bake at 375° F for 30 minutes or until a wooden pick inserted in center comes out clean. Cool 10 minutes in pan on a wire rack. Cut into squares. Garnish with powdered sugar, if desired. Serves 12. (*Note*: Makes a great snack cake for breakfast or brunch.)

Nutritional Information: 176 calories; 5.2g fat; 4.1g protein; 28.9g carbohydrate; 1.4g dietary fiber; 29mg cholesterol; 266mg sodium.

Member Survey

Please answer the following questions to help your leader plan your First Place 4 Health meetings so that your needs might be met in this session. Give this form to your leader at the first group meeting.

Name _____ Birth date _____

Please list those who live in your household.

Name	Relationship	Age

What church do you attend? _____

Are you interested in receiving more information about our church?

    Yes   No

Occupation _____

What talent or area of expertise would you be willing to share with our class?

_____

Why did you join First Place 4 Health?

_____

With notice, would you be willing to lead a Bible study discussion one week?

    Yes   No

Are you comfortable praying out loud? _____

If the assistant leader were absent, would you be willing to assist in weighing in members and possibly evaluating the Live It Trackers?

    Yes   No

Any other comments:

_____

_____

Personal Weight and Measurement Record

Week	Weight	+ or -	Goal this Session	Pounds to goal
1				
2				
3				
4				
5				
6				
7				
8				
9				
10				
11				
12				

Beginning Measurements

Waist _____ Hips _____ Thighs _____ Chest _____

Ending Measurements

Waist _____ Hips _____ Thighs _____ Chest _____

First Place 4 Health
Prayer Partner

MAKE EVERY DAY
YOUR BEST DAY
Week
1

SCRIPTURE VERSE TO MEMORIZE FOR WEEK TWO:
Forget the former things; do not dwell on the past.
ISAIAH 43:18

Date: _____

Name: _____

Home Phone: (____) _____

Work Phone: (____) _____

Email: _____

Personal Prayer Concerns:

_____
_____
_____
_____
_____
_____
_____

This form is for prayer requests that are personal to you and your journey in First Place 4 Health. Please complete this form and have it ready to turn in when you arrive at your group meeting.

First Place 4 Health
Prayer Partner

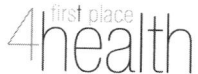

MAKE EVERY DAY
YOUR BEST DAY
Week
2

SCRIPTURE VERSE TO MEMORIZE FOR WEEK THREE:
Therefore do not worry about tomorrow, for tomorrow will worry about itself. Each day has enough trouble of its own.
MATTHEW 6:34

Date: _____

Name: _____

Home Phone: (_____) _____

Work Phone: (_____) _____

Email: _____

Personal Prayer Concerns:

_____
_____
_____
_____
_____
_____
_____
_____

This form is for prayer requests that are personal to you and your journey in First Place 4 Health. Please complete this form and have it ready to turn in when you arrive at your group meeting.

First Place 4 Health
Prayer Partner

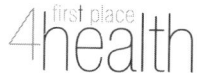

MAKE EVERY DAY
YOUR BEST DAY
Week
3

SCRIPTURE VERSE TO MEMORIZE FOR WEEK FOUR:
But I trust in you, O LORD; I say, "You are my God." My times are in your hands.
PSALM 31:14-15

Date: _____

Name: _____

Home Phone: (_____) _____

Work Phone: (_____) _____

Email: _____

Personal Prayer Concerns:

_____
_____
_____
_____
_____
_____
_____

This form is for prayer requests that are personal to you and your journey in First Place 4 Health. Please complete this form and have it ready to turn in when you arrive at your group meeting.

First Place 4 Health
Prayer Partner

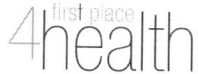

MAKE EVERY DAY
YOUR BEST DAY
Week
4

SCRIPTURE VERSE TO MEMORIZE FOR WEEK FIVE:
*The fear of the LORD is the beginning of wisdom;
all who follow his precepts have good understanding.*
PSALM 111:10

Date: _____

Name: _____

Home Phone: (_____) _____

Work Phone: (_____) _____

Email: _____

Personal Prayer Concerns:

_____
_____
_____
_____
_____
_____
_____

This form is for prayer requests that are personal to you and your journey in First Place 4 Health. Please complete this form and have it ready to turn in when you arrive at your group meeting.

First Place 4 Health
Prayer Partner

MAKE EVERY DAY
YOUR BEST DAY
Week
5

SCRIPTURE VERSE TO MEMORIZE FOR WEEK SIX:
A prudent man gives thought to his steps.
PROVERBS 14:15

Date: _____

Name: _____

Home Phone: (___) _____

Work Phone: (___) _____

Email: _____

Personal Prayer Concerns:

_____
_____
_____
_____
_____
_____
_____

This form is for prayer requests that are personal to you and your journey in First Place 4 Health. Please complete this form and have it ready to turn in when you arrive at your group meeting.

First Place 4 Health
Prayer Partner

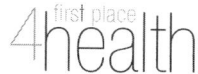

MAKE EVERY DAY
YOUR BEST DAY
Week
6

SCRIPTURE VERSE TO MEMORIZE FOR WEEK SEVEN:

He has made everything beautiful in its time. He has also set eternity in the hearts of men; yet they cannot fathom what God has done from beginning to end.

ECCLESIASTES 3:11

Date: _____

Name: _____

Home Phone: (_____) _____

Work Phone: (_____) _____

Email: _____

Personal Prayer Concerns:

_____
_____
_____
_____
_____
_____
_____
_____

This form is for prayer requests that are personal to you and your journey in First Place 4 Health. Please complete this form and have it ready to turn in when you arrive at your group meeting.

First Place 4 Health
Prayer Partner

MAKE EVERY DAY
YOUR BEST DAY
Week
7

SCRIPTURE VERSE TO MEMORIZE FOR WEEK EIGHT:

I will sing of the LORD's great love forever; with my mouth I will make your faithfulness known through all generations. I will declare that your love stands firm forever, that you established your faithfulness in heaven itself.

PSALM 89:1-2

Date: _____

Name: _____

Home Phone: (____) _____

Work Phone: (____) _____

Email: _____

Personal Prayer Concerns:

_____
_____
_____
_____
_____
_____
_____

This form is for prayer requests that are personal to you and your journey in First Place 4 Health. Please complete this form and have it ready to turn in when you arrive at your group meeting.

First Place 4 Health
Prayer Partner

MAKE EVERY DAY
YOUR BEST DAY
Week
8

SCRIPTURE VERSE TO MEMORIZE FOR WEEK NINE:

Train yourself to be godly. For physical training is of some value, but godliness has value for all things, holding promise for both the present life and the life to come.

1 TIMOTHY 4:7-8

Date: _____

Name: _____

Home Phone: (___) _____

Work Phone: (___) _____

Email: _____

Personal Prayer Concerns:

_____
_____
_____
_____
_____
_____
_____

This form is for prayer requests that are personal to you and your journey in First Place 4 Health. Please complete this form and have it ready to turn in when you arrive at your group meeting.

First Place 4 Health
Prayer Partner

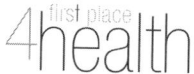

MAKE EVERY DAY
YOUR BEST DAY
Week
9

SCRIPTURE VERSE TO MEMORIZE FOR WEEK TEN:
We have this hope as an anchor for the soul, firm and secure.
HEBREWS 6:19

Date: _____

Name: _____

Home Phone: (_____) _____

Work Phone: (_____) _____

Email: _____

Personal Prayer Concerns:

_____
_____
_____
_____
_____
_____
_____
_____

This form is for prayer requests that are personal to you and your journey in First Place 4 Health. Please complete this form and have it ready to turn in when you arrive at your group meeting.

First Place 4 Health
Prayer Partner

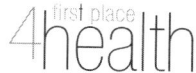

MAKE EVERY DAY
YOUR BEST DAY
Week
10

SCRIPTURE VERSE TO MEMORIZE FOR WEEK ELEVEN:

But just as you excel in everything—in faith, in speech, in knowledge, in complete earnestness and in your love for us—see that you also excel in this grace of giving.

2 CORINTHIANS 8:7

Date: _____

Name: _____

Home Phone: (____) _____

Work Phone: (____) _____

Email: _____

Personal Prayer Concerns:

_____
_____
_____
_____
_____
_____
_____

This form is for prayer requests that are personal to you and your journey in First Place 4 Health. Please complete this form and have it ready to turn in when you arrive at your group meeting.

First Place 4 Health
Prayer Partner

MAKE EVERY DAY
YOUR BEST DAY
Week
11

Date: _____

Name: _____

Home Phone: (____) _____

Work Phone: (____) _____

Email: _____

Personal Prayer Concerns:

_____
_____
_____
_____
_____
_____
_____

This form is for prayer requests that are personal to you and your journey in First Place 4 Health. Please complete this form and have it ready to turn in when you arrive at your group meeting.

Live It Tracker

Name: _____ Date: _____ Week #: ____

Loss/gain _____ lbs.   Calorie Range: _____   My food goal for the week: _____

Activity Level: None, < 30 min/day, 30-60 min/day, 60+ min/day   My activity goal for the week: _____
My spiritual goal for the week: _____

Group	Daily Calories							
	1300-1400	1500-1600	1700-1800	1900-2000	2100-2200	2300-2400	2500-2600	2700-2800
Fruits	1.5-2 c.	1.5-2 c.	1.5-2 c.	2-2.5 c.	2-2.5 c.	2.5-3.5 c.	3.5-4.5 c.	3.5-4.5 c.
Vegetables	1.5-2 c.	2-2.5 c.	2.5-3 c.	2.5-3 c.	3-3.5 c.	3.5-4.5 c.	4.5-5 c.	4.5-5 c.
Grains	5 oz-eq.	5-6 oz-eq.	6-7 oz-eq.	6-7 oz-eq.	7-8 oz-eq.	8-9 oz-eq.	9-10 oz-eq.	10-11 oz-eq.
Meat & Beans	4 oz-eq.	5 oz-eq.	5-5.5 oz-eq.	5.5-6.5 oz-eq.	6.5-7 oz-eq.	7-7.5 oz-eq.	7-7.5 oz-eq.	7.5-8 oz-eq.
Milk	2-3 c.	3 c.	3 c.	3 c.	3 c.	3 c.	3 c.	3 c.
Healthy Oils	4 tsp.	5 tsp.	5 tsp.	6 tsp.	6 tsp.	7 tsp.	8 tsp.	8 tsp.

Day/Date: ____

Breakfast: _____
Lunch: _____
Dinner: _____
Snacks: _____

GROUP	FRUITS	VEGETABLES	GRAINS	MEAT & BEANS	MILK	OILS
Goal Amount						
Estimate Your Total						
Total Calories						

Physical Activity: _____   Spiritual Activity: _____
Steps/Miles/Minutes: _____   My Emotions Today: ❏ Happy   ❏ Sad   ❏ Stressed

Day/Date: ____

Breakfast: _____
Lunch: _____
Dinner: _____
Snacks: _____

GROUP	FRUITS	VEGETABLES	GRAINS	MEAT & BEANS	MILK	OILS
Goal Amount						
Estimate Your Total						
Total Calories						

Physical Activity: _____   Spiritual Activity: _____
Steps/Miles/Minutes: _____   My Emotions Today: ❏ Happy   ❏ Sad   ❏ Stressed

Day/Date: ____

Breakfast: _____
Lunch: _____
Dinner: _____
Snacks: _____

GROUP	FRUITS	VEGETABLES	GRAINS	MEAT & BEANS	MILK	OILS
Goal Amount						
Estimate Your Total						
Total Calories						

Physical Activity: _____   Spiritual Activity: _____
Steps/Miles/Minutes: _____   My Emotions Today: ❏ Happy   ❏ Sad   ❏ Stressed

Copyright 2012 First Place 4 Health. Do not duplicate without permission from First Place 4 Health.

Day/Date: _____

Breakfast: _____
Lunch: _____
Dinner: _____
Snacks: _____

GROUP	FRUITS	VEGETABLES	GRAINS	MEAT & BEANS	MILK	OILS
Goal Amount						
Estimate Your Total						
Total Calories						

Physical Activity: _____ Spiritual Activity: _____
Steps/Miles/Minutes: _____ My Emotions Today: ❏ Happy ❏ Sad ❏ Stressed

---

Day/Date: _____

Breakfast: _____
Lunch: _____
Dinner: _____
Snacks: _____

GROUP	FRUITS	VEGETABLES	GRAINS	MEAT & BEANS	MILK	OILS
Goal Amount						
Estimate Your Total						
Total Calories						

Physical Activity: _____ Spiritual Activity: _____
Steps/Miles/Minutes: _____ My Emotions Today: ❏ Happy ❏ Sad ❏ Stressed

---

Day/Date: _____

Breakfast: _____
Lunch: _____
Dinner: _____
Snacks: _____

GROUP	FRUITS	VEGETABLES	GRAINS	MEAT & BEANS	MILK	OILS
Goal Amount						
Estimate Your Total						
Total Calories						

Physical Activity: _____ Spiritual Activity: _____
Steps/Miles/Minutes: _____ My Emotions Today: ❏ Happy ❏ Sad ❏ Stressed

---

Day/Date: _____

Breakfast: _____
Lunch: _____
Dinner: _____
Snacks: _____

GROUP	FRUITS	VEGETABLES	GRAINS	MEAT & BEANS	MILK	OILS
Goal Amount						
Estimate Your Total						
Total Calories						

Physical Activity: _____ Spiritual Activity: _____
Steps/Miles/Minutes: _____ My Emotions Today: ❏ Happy ❏ Sad ❏ Stressed

Live It Tracker

Name: _____ Date: _____ Week #: _____
Loss/gain _____ lbs. Calorie Range: _____ My food goal for the week: _____

Activity Level: None, < 30 min/day, 30-60 min/day, 60+ min/day   My activity goal for the week: _____
My spiritual goal for the week: _____

Group	Daily Calories							
	1300-1400	1500-1600	1700-1800	1900-2000	2100-2200	2300-2400	2500-2600	2700-2800
Fruits	1.5-2 c.	1.5-2 c.	1.5-2 c.	2-2.5 c.	2-2.5 c.	2.5-3.5 c.	3.5-4.5 c.	3.5-4.5 c.
Vegetables	1.5-2 c.	2-2.5 c.	2.5-3 c.	2.5-3 c.	3-3.5 c.	3.5-4.5 c.	4.5-5 c.	4.5-5 c.
Grains	5 oz-eq.	5-6 oz-eq.	6-7 oz-eq.	6-7 oz-eq.	7-8 oz-eq.	8-9 oz-eq.	9-10 oz-eq.	10-11 oz-eq.
Meat & Beans	4 oz-eq.	5 oz-eq.	5-5.5 oz-eq.	5.5-6.5 oz-eq.	6.5-7 oz-eq.	7-7.5 oz-eq.	7-7.5 oz-eq.	7.5-8 oz-eq.
Milk	2-3 c.	3 c.	3 c.	3 c.	3 c.	3 c.	3 c.	3 c.
Healthy Oils	4 tsp.	5 tsp.	5 tsp.	6 tsp.	6 tsp.	7 tsp.	8 tsp.	8 tsp.

Day/Date: _____

Breakfast: _____
Lunch: _____
Dinner: _____
Snacks: _____

GROUP	FRUITS	VEGETABLES	GRAINS	MEAT & BEANS	MILK	OILS
Goal Amount						
Estimate Your Total						
Total Calories						

Physical Activity: _____ Spiritual Activity: _____
Steps/Miles/Minutes: _____ My Emotions Today: ❏ Happy ❏ Sad ❏ Stressed

Day/Date: _____

Breakfast: _____
Lunch: _____
Dinner: _____
Snacks: _____

GROUP	FRUITS	VEGETABLES	GRAINS	MEAT & BEANS	MILK	OILS
Goal Amount						
Estimate Your Total						
Total Calories						

Physical Activity: _____ Spiritual Activity: _____
Steps/Miles/Minutes: _____ My Emotions Today: ❏ Happy ❏ Sad ❏ Stressed

Day/Date: _____

Breakfast: _____
Lunch: _____
Dinner: _____
Snacks: _____

GROUP	FRUITS	VEGETABLES	GRAINS	MEAT & BEANS	MILK	OILS
Goal Amount						
Estimate Your Total						
Total Calories						

Physical Activity: _____ Spiritual Activity: _____
Steps/Miles/Minutes: _____ My Emotions Today: ❏ Happy ❏ Sad ❏ Stressed

Day/Date:

Breakfast: _____
Lunch: _____
Dinner: _____
Snacks: _____

GROUP	FRUITS	VEGETABLES	GRAINS	MEAT & BEANS	MILK	OILS
Goal Amount						
Estimate Your Total						
Total Calories						

Physical Activity: _____ Spiritual Activity: _____
Steps/Miles/Minutes: _____ My Emotions Today: ❏ Happy ❏ Sad ❏ Stressed

---

Day/Date:

Breakfast: _____
Lunch: _____
Dinner: _____
Snacks: _____

GROUP	FRUITS	VEGETABLES	GRAINS	MEAT & BEANS	MILK	OILS
Goal Amount						
Estimate Your Total						
Total Calories						

Physical Activity: _____ Spiritual Activity: _____
Steps/Miles/Minutes: _____ My Emotions Today: ❏ Happy ❏ Sad ❏ Stressed

---

Day/Date:

Breakfast: _____
Lunch: _____
Dinner: _____
Snacks: _____

GROUP	FRUITS	VEGETABLES	GRAINS	MEAT & BEANS	MILK	OILS
Goal Amount						
Estimate Your Total						
Total Calories						

Physical Activity: _____ Spiritual Activity: _____
Steps/Miles/Minutes: _____ My Emotions Today: ❏ Happy ❏ Sad ❏ Stressed

---

Day/Date:

Breakfast: _____
Lunch: _____
Dinner: _____
Snacks: _____

GROUP	FRUITS	VEGETABLES	GRAINS	MEAT & BEANS	MILK	OILS
Goal Amount						
Estimate Your Total						
Total Calories						

Physical Activity: _____ Spiritual Activity: _____
Steps/Miles/Minutes: _____ My Emotions Today: ❏ Happy ❏ Sad ❏ Stressed

Live It Tracker

Name: _____ Date: _____ Week #: _____

Loss/gain _____ lbs. Calorie Range: _____ My food goal for the week: _____

Activity Level: None, < 30 min/day, 30-60 min/day, 60+ min/day My activity goal for the week: _____
My spiritual goal for the week: _____

Group	Daily Calories							
	1300-1400	1500-1600	1700-1800	1900-2000	2100-2200	2300-2400	2500-2600	2700-2800
Fruits	1.5-2 c.	1.5-2 c.	1.5-2 c.	2-2.5 c.	2-2.5 c.	2.5-3.5 c.	3.5-4.5 c.	3.5-4.5 c.
Vegetables	1.5-2 c.	2-2.5 c.	2.5-3 c.	2.5-3 c.	3-3.5 c.	3.5-4.5 c.	4.5-5 c.	4.5-5 c.
Grains	5 oz-eq.	5-6 oz-eq.	6-7 oz-eq.	6-7 oz-eq.	7-8 oz-eq.	8-9 oz-eq.	9-10 oz-eq.	10-11 oz-eq.
Meat & Beans	4 oz-eq.	5 oz-eq.	5-5.5 oz-eq.	5.5-6.5 oz-eq.	6.5-7 oz-eq.	7-7.5 oz-eq.	7-7.5 oz-eq.	7.5-8 oz-eq.
Milk	2-3 c.	3 c.	3 c.	3 c.	3 c.	3 c.	3 c.	3 c.
Healthy Oils	4 tsp.	5 tsp.	5 tsp.	6 tsp.	6 tsp.	7 tsp.	8 tsp.	8 tsp.

Day/Date: _____

Breakfast: _____
Lunch: _____
Dinner: _____
Snacks: _____

GROUP	FRUITS	VEGETABLES	GRAINS	MEAT & BEANS	MILK	OILS
Goal Amount						
Estimate Your Total						
Total Calories						

Physical Activity: _____ Spiritual Activity: _____
Steps/Miles/Minutes: _____ My Emotions Today: ❏ Happy ❏ Sad ❏ Stressed

---

Day/Date: _____

Breakfast: _____
Lunch: _____
Dinner: _____
Snacks: _____

GROUP	FRUITS	VEGETABLES	GRAINS	MEAT & BEANS	MILK	OILS
Goal Amount						
Estimate Your Total						
Total Calories						

Physical Activity: _____ Spiritual Activity: _____
Steps/Miles/Minutes: _____ My Emotions Today: ❏ Happy ❏ Sad ❏ Stressed

---

Day/Date: _____

Breakfast: _____
Lunch: _____
Dinner: _____
Snacks: _____

GROUP	FRUITS	VEGETABLES	GRAINS	MEAT & BEANS	MILK	OILS
Goal Amount						
Estimate Your Total						
Total Calories						

Physical Activity: _____ Spiritual Activity: _____
Steps/Miles/Minutes: _____ My Emotions Today: ❏ Happy ❏ Sad ❏ Stressed

Copyright 2012 First Place 4 Health. Do not duplicate without permission from First Place 4 Health.

Day/Date:

Breakfast: _____
Lunch: _____
Dinner: _____
Snacks: _____

GROUP	FRUITS	VEGETABLES	GRAINS	MEAT & BEANS	MILK	OILS
Goal Amount						
Estimate Your Total						
Total Calories						

Physical Activity: _____
Steps/Miles/Minutes: _____
Spiritual Activity: _____
My Emotions Today: ❏ Happy ❏ Sad ❏ Stressed

Day/Date:

Breakfast: _____
Lunch: _____
Dinner: _____
Snacks: _____

GROUP	FRUITS	VEGETABLES	GRAINS	MEAT & BEANS	MILK	OILS
Goal Amount						
Estimate Your Total						
Total Calories						

Physical Activity: _____
Steps/Miles/Minutes: _____
Spiritual Activity: _____
My Emotions Today: ❏ Happy ❏ Sad ❏ Stressed

Day/Date:

Breakfast: _____
Lunch: _____
Dinner: _____
Snacks: _____

GROUP	FRUITS	VEGETABLES	GRAINS	MEAT & BEANS	MILK	OILS
Goal Amount						
Estimate Your Total						
Total Calories						

Physical Activity: _____
Steps/Miles/Minutes: _____
Spiritual Activity: _____
My Emotions Today: ❏ Happy ❏ Sad ❏ Stressed

Day/Date:

Breakfast: _____
Lunch: _____
Dinner: _____
Snacks: _____

GROUP	FRUITS	VEGETABLES	GRAINS	MEAT & BEANS	MILK	OILS
Goal Amount						
Estimate Your Total						
Total Calories						

Physical Activity: _____
Steps/Miles/Minutes: _____
Spiritual Activity: _____
My Emotions Today: ❏ Happy ❏ Sad ❏ Stressed

Live It Tracker

Name: _____ Date: _____ Week #: _____

Loss/gain _____ lbs.   Calorie Range: _____   My food goal for the week: _____

Activity Level: None, < 30 min/day, 30-60 min/day, 60+ min/day   My activity goal for the week: _____
My spiritual goal for the week: _____

Group	Daily Calories							
	1300-1400	1500-1600	1700-1800	1900-2000	2100-2200	2300-2400	2500-2600	2700-2800
Fruits	1.5-2 c.	1.5-2 c.	1.5-2 c.	2-2.5 c.	2-2.5 c.	2.5-3.5 c.	3.5-4.5 c.	3.5-4.5 c.
Vegetables	1.5-2 c.	2-2.5 c.	2.5-3 c.	2.5-3 c.	3-3.5 c.	3.5-4.5 c.	4.5-5 c.	4.5-5 c.
Grains	5 oz-eq.	5-6 oz-eq.	6-7 oz-eq.	6-7 oz-eq.	7-8 oz-eq.	8-9 oz-eq.	9-10 oz-eq.	10-11 oz-eq.
Meat & Beans	4 oz-eq.	5 oz-eq.	5-5.5 oz-eq.	5.5-6.5 oz-eq.	6.5-7 oz-eq.	7-7.5 oz-eq.	7-7.5 oz-eq.	7.5-8 oz-eq.
Milk	2-3 c.	3 c.	3 c.	3 c.	3 c.	3 c.	3 c.	3 c.
Healthy Oils	4 tsp.	5 tsp.	5 tsp.	6 tsp.	6 tsp.	7 tsp.	8 tsp.	8 tsp.

Day/Date:

Breakfast: _____
Lunch: _____
Dinner: _____
Snacks: _____

GROUP	FRUITS	VEGETABLES	GRAINS	MEAT & BEANS	MILK	OILS
Goal Amount						
Estimate Your Total						
Total Calories						

Physical Activity: _____ Spiritual Activity: _____
Steps/Miles/Minutes: _____ My Emotions Today: ❏ Happy   ❏ Sad   ❏ Stressed

---

Day/Date:

Breakfast: _____
Lunch: _____
Dinner: _____
Snacks: _____

GROUP	FRUITS	VEGETABLES	GRAINS	MEAT & BEANS	MILK	OILS
Goal Amount						
Estimate Your Total						
Total Calories						

Physical Activity: _____ Spiritual Activity: _____
Steps/Miles/Minutes: _____ My Emotions Today: ❏ Happy   ❏ Sad   ❏ Stressed

---

Day/Date:

Breakfast: _____
Lunch: _____
Dinner: _____
Snacks: _____

GROUP	FRUITS	VEGETABLES	GRAINS	MEAT & BEANS	MILK	OILS
Goal Amount						
Estimate Your Total						
Total Calories						

Physical Activity: _____ Spiritual Activity: _____
Steps/Miles/Minutes: _____ My Emotions Today: ❏ Happy   ❏ Sad   ❏ Stressed

Copyright 2012 First Place 4 Health. Do not duplicate without permission from First Place 4 Health.

Day/Date: _____

Breakfast: _____
Lunch: _____
Dinner: _____
Snacks: _____

GROUP	FRUITS	VEGETABLES	GRAINS	MEAT & BEANS	MILK	OILS
Goal Amount						
Estimate Your Total						
Total Calories						

Physical Activity: _____ Spiritual Activity: _____
Steps/Miles/Minutes: _____ My Emotions Today: ❑ Happy ❑ Sad ❑ Stressed

---

Day/Date: _____

Breakfast: _____
Lunch: _____
Dinner: _____
Snacks: _____

GROUP	FRUITS	VEGETABLES	GRAINS	MEAT & BEANS	MILK	OILS
Goal Amount						
Estimate Your Total						
Total Calories						

Physical Activity: _____ Spiritual Activity: _____
Steps/Miles/Minutes: _____ My Emotions Today: ❑ Happy ❑ Sad ❑ Stressed

---

Day/Date: _____

Breakfast: _____
Lunch: _____
Dinner: _____
Snacks: _____

GROUP	FRUITS	VEGETABLES	GRAINS	MEAT & BEANS	MILK	OILS
Goal Amount						
Estimate Your Total						
Total Calories						

Physical Activity: _____ Spiritual Activity: _____
Steps/Miles/Minutes: _____ My Emotions Today: ❑ Happy ❑ Sad ❑ Stressed

---

Day/Date: _____

Breakfast: _____
Lunch: _____
Dinner: _____
Snacks: _____

GROUP	FRUITS	VEGETABLES	GRAINS	MEAT & BEANS	MILK	OILS
Goal Amount						
Estimate Your Total						
Total Calories						

Physical Activity: _____ Spiritual Activity: _____
Steps/Miles/Minutes: _____ My Emotions Today: ❑ Happy ❑ Sad ❑ Stressed

Live It Tracker

Name: _____ Date: _____ Week #: _____

Loss/gain _____ lbs.   Calorie Range: _____   My food goal for the week: _____

Activity Level: None, < 30 min/day, 30-60 min/day, 60+ min/day   My activity goal for the week: _____

My spiritual goal for the week: _____

Group	Daily Calories							
	1300-1400	1500-1600	1700-1800	1900-2000	2100-2200	2300-2400	2500-2600	2700-2800
Fruits	1.5-2 c.	1.5-2 c.	1.5-2 c.	2-2.5 c.	2-2.5 c.	2.5-3.5 c.	3.5-4.5 c.	3.5-4.5 c.
Vegetables	1.5-2 c.	2-2.5 c.	2.5-3 c.	2.5-3 c.	3-3.5 c.	3.5-4.5 c.	4.5-5 c.	4.5-5 c.
Grains	5 oz-eq.	5-6 oz-eq.	6-7 oz-eq.	6-7 oz-eq.	7-8 oz-eq.	8-9 oz-eq.	9-10 oz-eq.	10-11 oz-eq.
Meat & Beans	4 oz-eq.	5 oz-eq.	5-5.5 oz-eq.	5.5-6.5 oz-eq.	6.5-7 oz-eq.	7-7.5 oz-eq.	7-7.5 oz-eq.	7.5-8 oz-eq.
Milk	2-3 c.	3 c.	3 c.	3 c.	3 c.	3 c.	3 c.	3 c.
Healthy Oils	4 tsp.	5 tsp.	5 tsp.	6 tsp.	6 tsp.	7 tsp.	8 tsp.	8 tsp.

Day/Date: _____

Breakfast: _____
Lunch: _____
Dinner: _____
Snacks: _____

GROUP	FRUITS	VEGETABLES	GRAINS	MEAT & BEANS	MILK	OILS
Goal Amount						
Estimate Your Total						
Total Calories						

Physical Activity: _____   Spiritual Activity: _____
Steps/Miles/Minutes: _____   My Emotions Today: ❏ Happy   ❏ Sad   ❏ Stressed

Day/Date: _____

Breakfast: _____
Lunch: _____
Dinner: _____
Snacks: _____

GROUP	FRUITS	VEGETABLES	GRAINS	MEAT & BEANS	MILK	OILS
Goal Amount						
Estimate Your Total						
Total Calories						

Physical Activity: _____   Spiritual Activity: _____
Steps/Miles/Minutes: _____   My Emotions Today: ❏ Happy   ❏ Sad   ❏ Stressed

Day/Date: _____

Breakfast: _____
Lunch: _____
Dinner: _____
Snacks: _____

GROUP	FRUITS	VEGETABLES	GRAINS	MEAT & BEANS	MILK	OILS
Goal Amount						
Estimate Your Total						
Total Calories						

Physical Activity: _____   Spiritual Activity: _____
Steps/Miles/Minutes: _____   My Emotions Today: ❏ Happy   ❏ Sad   ❏ Stressed

Copyright 2012 First Place 4 Health. Do not duplicate without permission from First Place 4 Health.

Day/Date:

Breakfast: _____
Lunch: _____
Dinner: _____
Snacks: _____

GROUP	FRUITS	VEGETABLES	GRAINS	MEAT & BEANS	MILK	OILS
Goal Amount						
Estimate Your Total						
Total Calories						

Physical Activity: _____ Spiritual Activity: _____
Steps/Miles/Minutes: _____ My Emotions Today: ❏ Happy ❏ Sad ❏ Stressed

---

Day/Date:

Breakfast: _____
Lunch: _____
Dinner: _____
Snacks: _____

GROUP	FRUITS	VEGETABLES	GRAINS	MEAT & BEANS	MILK	OILS
Goal Amount						
Estimate Your Total						
Total Calories						

Physical Activity: _____ Spiritual Activity: _____
Steps/Miles/Minutes: _____ My Emotions Today: ❏ Happy ❏ Sad ❏ Stressed

---

Day/Date:

Breakfast: _____
Lunch: _____
Dinner: _____
Snacks: _____

GROUP	FRUITS	VEGETABLES	GRAINS	MEAT & BEANS	MILK	OILS
Goal Amount						
Estimate Your Total						
Total Calories						

Physical Activity: _____ Spiritual Activity: _____
Steps/Miles/Minutes: _____ My Emotions Today: ❏ Happy ❏ Sad ❏ Stressed

---

Day/Date:

Breakfast: _____
Lunch: _____
Dinner: _____
Snacks: _____

GROUP	FRUITS	VEGETABLES	GRAINS	MEAT & BEANS	MILK	OILS
Goal Amount						
Estimate Your Total						
Total Calories						

Physical Activity: _____ Spiritual Activity: _____
Steps/Miles/Minutes: _____ My Emotions Today: ❏ Happy ❏ Sad ❏ Stressed

Live It Tracker

Name: _____ Date: _____ Week #: _____
Loss/gain _____ lbs. Calorie Range: _____ My food goal for the week: _____

Activity Level: None, < 30 min/day, 30-60 min/day, 60+ min/day My activity goal for the week: _____
My spiritual goal for the week: _____

Group	Daily Calories							
	1300-1400	1500-1600	1700-1800	1900-2000	2100-2200	2300-2400	2500-2600	2700-2800
Fruits	1.5-2 c.	1.5-2 c.	1.5-2 c.	2-2.5 c.	2-2.5 c.	2.5-3.5 c.	3.5-4.5 c.	3.5-4.5 c.
Vegetables	1.5-2 c.	2-2.5 c.	2.5-3 c.	2.5-3 c.	3-3.5 c.	3.5-4.5 c.	4.5-5 c.	4.5-5 c.
Grains	5 oz-eq.	5-6 oz-eq.	6-7 oz-eq.	6-7 oz-eq.	7-8 oz-eq.	8-9 oz-eq.	9-10 oz-eq.	10-11 oz-eq.
Meat & Beans	4 oz-eq.	5 oz-eq.	5-5.5 oz-eq.	5.5-6.5 oz-eq.	6.5-7 oz-eq.	7-7.5 oz-eq.	7-7.5 oz-eq.	7.5-8 oz-eq.
Milk	2-3 c.	3 c.	3 c.	3 c.	3 c.	3 c.	3 c.	3 c.
Healthy Oils	4 tsp.	5 tsp.	5 tsp.	6 tsp.	6 tsp.	7 tsp.	8 tsp.	8 tsp.

Day/Date: _____

Breakfast: _____
Lunch: _____
Dinner: _____
Snacks: _____

GROUP	FRUITS	VEGETABLES	GRAINS	MEAT & BEANS	MILK	OILS
Goal Amount						
Estimate Your Total						
Total Calories						

Physical Activity: _____ Spiritual Activity: _____
Steps/Miles/Minutes: _____ My Emotions Today: ❏ Happy   ❏ Sad   ❏ Stressed

Day/Date: _____

Breakfast: _____
Lunch: _____
Dinner: _____
Snacks: _____

GROUP	FRUITS	VEGETABLES	GRAINS	MEAT & BEANS	MILK	OILS
Goal Amount						
Estimate Your Total						
Total Calories						

Physical Activity: _____ Spiritual Activity: _____
Steps/Miles/Minutes: _____ My Emotions Today: ❏ Happy   ❏ Sad   ❏ Stressed

Day/Date: _____

Breakfast: _____
Lunch: _____
Dinner: _____
Snacks: _____

GROUP	FRUITS	VEGETABLES	GRAINS	MEAT & BEANS	MILK	OILS
Goal Amount						
Estimate Your Total						
Total Calories						

Physical Activity: _____ Spiritual Activity: _____
Steps/Miles/Minutes: _____ My Emotions Today: ❏ Happy   ❏ Sad   ❏ Stressed

Copyright 2012 First Place 4 Health. Do not duplicate without permission from First Place 4 Health.

Day/Date: ___

Breakfast: _____
Lunch: _____
Dinner: _____
Snacks: _____

GROUP	FRUITS	VEGETABLES	GRAINS	MEAT & BEANS	MILK	OILS
Goal Amount						
Estimate Your Total						
Total Calories						

Physical Activity: _____
Steps/Miles/Minutes: _____
Spiritual Activity: _____
My Emotions Today: ❏ Happy ❏ Sad ❏ Stressed

Day/Date: ___

Breakfast: _____
Lunch: _____
Dinner: _____
Snacks: _____

GROUP	FRUITS	VEGETABLES	GRAINS	MEAT & BEANS	MILK	OILS
Goal Amount						
Estimate Your Total						
Total Calories						

Physical Activity: _____
Steps/Miles/Minutes: _____
Spiritual Activity: _____
My Emotions Today: ❏ Happy ❏ Sad ❏ Stressed

Day/Date: ___

Breakfast: _____
Lunch: _____
Dinner: _____
Snacks: _____

GROUP	FRUITS	VEGETABLES	GRAINS	MEAT & BEANS	MILK	OILS
Goal Amount						
Estimate Your Total						
Total Calories						

Physical Activity: _____
Steps/Miles/Minutes: _____
Spiritual Activity: _____
My Emotions Today: ❏ Happy ❏ Sad ❏ Stressed

Day/Date: ___

Breakfast: _____
Lunch: _____
Dinner: _____
Snacks: _____

GROUP	FRUITS	VEGETABLES	GRAINS	MEAT & BEANS	MILK	OILS
Goal Amount						
Estimate Your Total						
Total Calories						

Physical Activity: _____
Steps/Miles/Minutes: _____
Spiritual Activity: _____
My Emotions Today: ❏ Happy ❏ Sad ❏ Stressed

Copyright 2012 First Place 4 Health. Do not duplicate without permission from First Place 4 Health.

Live It Tracker

Name: _____ Date: _____ Week #: _____
Loss/gain _____ lbs.   Calorie Range: _____   My food goal for the week: _____

Activity Level: None, < 30 min/day, 30-60 min/day, 60+ min/day   My activity goal for the week: _____
My spiritual goal for the week: _____

Group	Daily Calories							
	1300-1400	1500-1600	1700-1800	1900-2000	2100-2200	2300-2400	2500-2600	2700-2800
Fruits	1.5-2 c.	1.5-2 c.	1.5-2 c.	2-2.5 c.	2-2.5 c.	2.5-3.5 c.	3.5-4.5 c.	3.5-4.5 c.
Vegetables	1.5-2 c.	2-2.5 c.	2.5-3 c.	2.5-3 c.	3-3.5 c.	3.5-4.5 c.	4.5-5 c.	4.5-5 c.
Grains	5 oz-eq.	5-6 oz-eq.	6-7 oz-eq.	6-7 oz-eq.	7-8 oz-eq.	8-9 oz-eq.	9-10 oz-eq.	10-11 oz-eq.
Meat & Beans	4 oz-eq.	5 oz-eq.	5-5.5 oz-eq.	5.5-6.5 oz-eq.	6.5-7 oz-eq.	7-7.5 oz-eq.	7-7.5 oz-eq.	7.5-8 oz-eq.
Milk	2-3 c.	3 c.	3 c.	3 c.	3 c.	3 c.	3 c.	3 c.
Healthy Oils	4 tsp.	5 tsp.	5 tsp.	6 tsp.	6 tsp.	7 tsp.	8 tsp.	8 tsp.

Day/Date: _____

Breakfast: _____
Lunch: _____
Dinner: _____
Snacks: _____

GROUP	FRUITS	VEGETABLES	GRAINS	MEAT & BEANS	MILK	OILS
Goal Amount						
Estimate Your Total						
Total Calories						

Physical Activity: _____ Spiritual Activity: _____
Steps/Miles/Minutes: _____   My Emotions Today: ❏ Happy ❏ Sad ❏ Stressed

Day/Date: _____

Breakfast: _____
Lunch: _____
Dinner: _____
Snacks: _____

GROUP	FRUITS	VEGETABLES	GRAINS	MEAT & BEANS	MILK	OILS
Goal Amount						
Estimate Your Total						
Total Calories						

Physical Activity: _____ Spiritual Activity: _____
Steps/Miles/Minutes: _____   My Emotions Today: ❏ Happy ❏ Sad ❏ Stressed

Day/Date: _____

Breakfast: _____
Lunch: _____
Dinner: _____
Snacks: _____

GROUP	FRUITS	VEGETABLES	GRAINS	MEAT & BEANS	MILK	OILS
Goal Amount						
Estimate Your Total						
Total Calories						

Physical Activity: _____ Spiritual Activity: _____
Steps/Miles/Minutes: _____   My Emotions Today: ❏ Happy ❏ Sad ❏ Stressed

Copyright 2012 First Place 4 Health. Do not duplicate without permission from First Place 4 Health.

Day/Date:

Breakfast: _____
Lunch: _____
Dinner: _____
Snacks: _____

GROUP	FRUITS	VEGETABLES	GRAINS	MEAT & BEANS	MILK	OILS
Goal Amount						
Estimate Your Total						
Total Calories						

Physical Activity: _____ Spiritual Activity: _____
Steps/Miles/Minutes: _____ My Emotions Today: ❏ Happy ❏ Sad ❏ Stressed

---

Day/Date:

Breakfast: _____
Lunch: _____
Dinner: _____
Snacks: _____

GROUP	FRUITS	VEGETABLES	GRAINS	MEAT & BEANS	MILK	OILS
Goal Amount						
Estimate Your Total						
Total Calories						

Physical Activity: _____ Spiritual Activity: _____
Steps/Miles/Minutes: _____ My Emotions Today: ❏ Happy ❏ Sad ❏ Stressed

---

Day/Date:

Breakfast: _____
Lunch: _____
Dinner: _____
Snacks: _____

GROUP	FRUITS	VEGETABLES	GRAINS	MEAT & BEANS	MILK	OILS
Goal Amount						
Estimate Your Total						
Total Calories						

Physical Activity: _____ Spiritual Activity: _____
Steps/Miles/Minutes: _____ My Emotions Today: ❏ Happy ❏ Sad ❏ Stressed

---

Day/Date:

Breakfast: _____
Lunch: _____
Dinner: _____
Snacks: _____

GROUP	FRUITS	VEGETABLES	GRAINS	MEAT & BEANS	MILK	OILS
Goal Amount						
Estimate Your Total						
Total Calories						

Physical Activity: _____ Spiritual Activity: _____
Steps/Miles/Minutes: _____ My Emotions Today: ❏ Happy ❏ Sad ❏ Stressed

Live It Tracker

Name: _____ Date: _____ Week #: ____

Loss/gain _____ lbs.   Calorie Range: _____   My food goal for the week: _____

Activity Level: None, < 30 min/day, 30-60 min/day, 60+ min/day   My activity goal for the week: _____

My spiritual goal for the week: _____

Group	Daily Calories							
	1300-1400	1500-1600	1700-1800	1900-2000	2100-2200	2300-2400	2500-2600	2700-2800
Fruits	1.5-2 c.	1.5-2 c.	1.5-2 c.	2-2.5 c.	2-2.5 c.	2.5-3.5 c.	3.5-4.5 c.	3.5-4.5 c.
Vegetables	1.5-2 c.	2-2.5 c.	2.5-3 c.	2.5-3 c.	3-3.5 c.	3.5-4.5 c.	4.5-5 c.	4.5-5 c.
Grains	5 oz-eq.	5-6 oz-eq.	6-7 oz-eq.	6-7 oz-eq.	7-8 oz-eq.	8-9 oz-eq.	9-10 oz-eq.	10-11 oz-eq.
Meat & Beans	4 oz-eq.	5 oz-eq.	5-5.5 oz-eq.	5.5-6.5 oz-eq.	6.5-7 oz-eq.	7-7.5 oz-eq.	7-7.5 oz-eq.	7.5-8 oz-eq.
Milk	2-3 c.	3 c.	3 c.	3 c.	3 c.	3 c.	3 c.	3 c.
Healthy Oils	4 tsp.	5 tsp.	5 tsp.	6 tsp.	6 tsp.	7 tsp.	8 tsp.	8 tsp.

Day/Date:

Breakfast: _____
Lunch: _____
Dinner: _____
Snacks: _____

GROUP	FRUITS	VEGETABLES	GRAINS	MEAT & BEANS	MILK	OILS
Goal Amount						
Estimate Your Total						
Total Calories						

Physical Activity: _____   Spiritual Activity: _____
Steps/Miles/Minutes: _____   My Emotions Today: ☐ Happy ☐ Sad ☐ Stressed

Day/Date:

Breakfast: _____
Lunch: _____
Dinner: _____
Snacks: _____

GROUP	FRUITS	VEGETABLES	GRAINS	MEAT & BEANS	MILK	OILS
Goal Amount						
Estimate Your Total						
Total Calories						

Physical Activity: _____   Spiritual Activity: _____
Steps/Miles/Minutes: _____   My Emotions Today: ☐ Happy ☐ Sad ☐ Stressed

Day/Date:

Breakfast: _____
Lunch: _____
Dinner: _____
Snacks: _____

GROUP	FRUITS	VEGETABLES	GRAINS	MEAT & BEANS	MILK	OILS
Goal Amount						
Estimate Your Total						
Total Calories						

Physical Activity: _____   Spiritual Activity: _____
Steps/Miles/Minutes: _____   My Emotions Today: ☐ Happy ☐ Sad ☐ Stressed

Copyright 2012 First Place 4 Health. Do not duplicate without permission from First Place 4 Health.

Day/Date:

Breakfast: _____
Lunch: _____
Dinner: _____
Snacks: _____

GROUP	FRUITS	VEGETABLES	GRAINS	MEAT & BEANS	MILK	OILS
Goal Amount						
Estimate Your Total						
Total Calories						

Physical Activity: _____
Steps/Miles/Minutes: _____
Spiritual Activity: _____
My Emotions Today: ❏ Happy ❏ Sad ❏ Stressed

Day/Date:

Breakfast: _____
Lunch: _____
Dinner: _____
Snacks: _____

GROUP	FRUITS	VEGETABLES	GRAINS	MEAT & BEANS	MILK	OILS
Goal Amount						
Estimate Your Total						
Total Calories						

Physical Activity: _____
Steps/Miles/Minutes: _____
Spiritual Activity: _____
My Emotions Today: ❏ Happy ❏ Sad ❏ Stressed

Day/Date:

Breakfast: _____
Lunch: _____
Dinner: _____
Snacks: _____

GROUP	FRUITS	VEGETABLES	GRAINS	MEAT & BEANS	MILK	OILS
Goal Amount						
Estimate Your Total						
Total Calories						

Physical Activity: _____
Steps/Miles/Minutes: _____
Spiritual Activity: _____
My Emotions Today: ❏ Happy ❏ Sad ❏ Stressed

Day/Date:

Breakfast: _____
Lunch: _____
Dinner: _____
Snacks: _____

GROUP	FRUITS	VEGETABLES	GRAINS	MEAT & BEANS	MILK	OILS
Goal Amount						
Estimate Your Total						
Total Calories						

Physical Activity: _____
Steps/Miles/Minutes: _____
Spiritual Activity: _____
My Emotions Today: ❏ Happy ❏ Sad ❏ Stressed

Copyright 2012 First Place 4 Health. Do not duplicate without permission from First Place 4 Health.

Live It Tracker

Name: _____ Date: _____ Week #: _____

Loss/gain _____ lbs. Calorie Range: _____ My food goal for the week: _____

Activity Level: None, < 30 min/day, 30-60 min/day, 60+ min/day   My activity goal for the week: _____
My spiritual goal for the week: _____

Group	Daily Calories							
	1300-1400	1500-1600	1700-1800	1900-2000	2100-2200	2300-2400	2500-2600	2700-2800
Fruits	1.5-2 c.	1.5-2 c.	1.5-2 c.	2-2.5 c.	2-2.5 c.	2.5-3.5 c.	3.5-4.5 c.	3.5-4.5 c.
Vegetables	1.5-2 c.	2-2.5 c.	2.5-3 c.	2.5-3 c.	3-3.5 c.	3.5-4.5 c.	4.5-5 c.	4.5-5 c.
Grains	5 oz-eq.	5-6 oz-eq.	6-7 oz-eq.	6-7 oz-eq.	7-8 oz-eq.	8-9 oz-eq.	9-10 oz-eq.	10-11 oz-eq.
Meat & Beans	4 oz-eq.	5 oz-eq.	5-5.5 oz-eq.	5.5-6.5 oz-eq.	6.5-7 oz-eq.	7-7.5 oz-eq.	7-7.5 oz-eq.	7.5-8 oz-eq.
Milk	2-3 c.	3 c.	3 c.	3 c.	3 c.	3 c.	3 c.	3 c.
Healthy Oils	4 tsp.	5 tsp.	5 tsp.	6 tsp.	6 tsp.	7 tsp.	8 tsp.	8 tsp.

Day/Date: _____

Breakfast: _____
Lunch: _____
Dinner: _____
Snacks: _____

GROUP	FRUITS	VEGETABLES	GRAINS	MEAT & BEANS	MILK	OILS
Goal Amount						
Estimate Your Total						
Total Calories						

Physical Activity: _____ Spiritual Activity: _____
Steps/Miles/Minutes: _____ My Emotions Today: ❑ Happy ❑ Sad ❑ Stressed

Day/Date: _____

Breakfast: _____
Lunch: _____
Dinner: _____
Snacks: _____

GROUP	FRUITS	VEGETABLES	GRAINS	MEAT & BEANS	MILK	OILS
Goal Amount						
Estimate Your Total						
Total Calories						

Physical Activity: _____ Spiritual Activity: _____
Steps/Miles/Minutes: _____ My Emotions Today: ❑ Happy ❑ Sad ❑ Stressed

Day/Date: _____

Breakfast: _____
Lunch: _____
Dinner: _____
Snacks: _____

GROUP	FRUITS	VEGETABLES	GRAINS	MEAT & BEANS	MILK	OILS
Goal Amount						
Estimate Your Total						
Total Calories						

Physical Activity: _____ Spiritual Activity: _____
Steps/Miles/Minutes: _____ My Emotions Today: ❑ Happy ❑ Sad ❑ Stressed

Copyright 2012 First Place 4 Health. Do not duplicate without permission from First Place 4 Health.

Day/Date: ___

Breakfast: ___
Lunch: ___
Dinner: ___
Snacks: ___

GROUP	FRUITS	VEGETABLES	GRAINS	MEAT & BEANS	MILK	OILS
Goal Amount						
Estimate Your Total						
Total Calories						

Physical Activity: ___
Steps/Miles/Minutes: ___
Spiritual Activity: ___
My Emotions Today: ❏ Happy ❏ Sad ❏ Stressed

Day/Date: ___

Breakfast: ___
Lunch: ___
Dinner: ___
Snacks: ___

GROUP	FRUITS	VEGETABLES	GRAINS	MEAT & BEANS	MILK	OILS
Goal Amount						
Estimate Your Total						
Total Calories						

Physical Activity: ___
Steps/Miles/Minutes: ___
Spiritual Activity: ___
My Emotions Today: ❏ Happy ❏ Sad ❏ Stressed

Day/Date: ___

Breakfast: ___
Lunch: ___
Dinner: ___
Snacks: ___

GROUP	FRUITS	VEGETABLES	GRAINS	MEAT & BEANS	MILK	OILS
Goal Amount						
Estimate Your Total						
Total Calories						

Physical Activity: ___
Steps/Miles/Minutes: ___
Spiritual Activity: ___
My Emotions Today: ❏ Happy ❏ Sad ❏ Stressed

Day/Date: ___

Breakfast: ___
Lunch: ___
Dinner: ___
Snacks: ___

GROUP	FRUITS	VEGETABLES	GRAINS	MEAT & BEANS	MILK	OILS
Goal Amount						
Estimate Your Total						
Total Calories						

Physical Activity: ___
Steps/Miles/Minutes: ___
Spiritual Activity: ___
My Emotions Today: ❏ Happy ❏ Sad ❏ Stressed

Live It Tracker

Name: _____ Date: _____ Week #: _____

Loss/gain _____ lbs.   Calorie Range: _____   My food goal for the week: _____

Activity Level: None, < 30 min/day, 30-60 min/day, 60+ min/day   My activity goal for the week: _____

My spiritual goal for the week: _____

Group	Daily Calories							
	1300-1400	1500-1600	1700-1800	1900-2000	2100-2200	2300-2400	2500-2600	2700-2800
Fruits	1.5-2 c.	1.5-2 c.	1.5-2 c.	2-2.5 c.	2-2.5 c.	2.5-3.5 c.	3.5-4.5 c.	3.5-4.5 c.
Vegetables	1.5-2 c.	2-2.5 c.	2.5-3 c.	2.5-3 c.	3-3.5 c.	3.5-4.5 c.	4.5-5 c.	4.5-5 c.
Grains	5 oz-eq.	5-6 oz-eq.	6-7 oz-eq.	6-7 oz-eq.	7-8 oz-eq.	8-9 oz-eq.	9-10 oz-eq.	10-11 oz-eq.
Meat & Beans	4 oz-eq.	5 oz-eq.	5-5.5 oz-eq.	5.5-6.5 oz-eq.	6.5-7 oz-eq.	7-7.5 oz-eq.	7-7.5 oz-eq.	7.5-8 oz-eq.
Milk	2-3 c.	3 c.	3 c.	3 c.	3 c.	3 c.	3 c.	3 c.
Healthy Oils	4 tsp.	5 tsp.	5 tsp.	6 tsp.	6 tsp.	7 tsp.	8 tsp.	8 tsp.

Day/Date: _____

Breakfast: _____
Lunch: _____
Dinner: _____
Snacks: _____

GROUP	FRUITS	VEGETABLES	GRAINS	MEAT & BEANS	MILK	OILS
Goal Amount						
Estimate Your Total						
Total Calories						

Physical Activity: _____   Spiritual Activity: _____
Steps/Miles/Minutes: _____   My Emotions Today: ❏ Happy ❏ Sad ❏ Stressed

Day/Date: _____

Breakfast: _____
Lunch: _____
Dinner: _____
Snacks: _____

GROUP	FRUITS	VEGETABLES	GRAINS	MEAT & BEANS	MILK	OILS
Goal Amount						
Estimate Your Total						
Total Calories						

Physical Activity: _____   Spiritual Activity: _____
Steps/Miles/Minutes: _____   My Emotions Today: ❏ Happy ❏ Sad ❏ Stressed

Day/Date: _____

Breakfast: _____
Lunch: _____
Dinner: _____
Snacks: _____

GROUP	FRUITS	VEGETABLES	GRAINS	MEAT & BEANS	MILK	OILS
Goal Amount						
Estimate Your Total						
Total Calories						

Physical Activity: _____   Spiritual Activity: _____
Steps/Miles/Minutes: _____   My Emotions Today: ❏ Happy ❏ Sad ❏ Stressed

Copyright 2012 First Place 4 Health. Do not duplicate without permission from First Place 4 Health.

Day/Date:

Breakfast: _____
Lunch: _____
Dinner: _____
Snacks: _____

GROUP	FRUITS	VEGETABLES	GRAINS	MEAT & BEANS	MILK	OILS
Goal Amount						
Estimate Your Total						
Total Calories						

Physical Activity: _____
Steps/Miles/Minutes: _____
Spiritual Activity: _____
My Emotions Today: ❏ Happy ❏ Sad ❏ Stressed

Day/Date:

Breakfast: _____
Lunch: _____
Dinner: _____
Snacks: _____

GROUP	FRUITS	VEGETABLES	GRAINS	MEAT & BEANS	MILK	OILS
Goal Amount						
Estimate Your Total						
Total Calories						

Physical Activity: _____
Steps/Miles/Minutes: _____
Spiritual Activity: _____
My Emotions Today: ❏ Happy ❏ Sad ❏ Stressed

Day/Date:

Breakfast: _____
Lunch: _____
Dinner: _____
Snacks: _____

GROUP	FRUITS	VEGETABLES	GRAINS	MEAT & BEANS	MILK	OILS
Goal Amount						
Estimate Your Total						
Total Calories						

Physical Activity: _____
Steps/Miles/Minutes: _____
Spiritual Activity: _____
My Emotions Today: ❏ Happy ❏ Sad ❏ Stressed

Day/Date:

Breakfast: _____
Lunch: _____
Dinner: _____
Snacks: _____

GROUP	FRUITS	VEGETABLES	GRAINS	MEAT & BEANS	MILK	OILS
Goal Amount						
Estimate Your Total						
Total Calories						

Physical Activity: _____
Steps/Miles/Minutes: _____
Spiritual Activity: _____
My Emotions Today: ❏ Happy ❏ Sad ❏ Stressed

Live It Tracker

Name: _____ Date: _____ Week #: _____
Loss/gain _____ lbs. Calorie Range: _____ My food goal for the week: _____

Activity Level: None, < 30 min/day, 30-60 min/day, 60+ min/day My activity goal for the week: _____
My spiritual goal for the week: _____

Group	Daily Calories							
	1300-1400	1500-1600	1700-1800	1900-2000	2100-2200	2300-2400	2500-2600	2700-2800
Fruits	1.5-2 c.	1.5-2 c.	1.5-2 c.	2-2.5 c.	2-2.5 c.	2.5-3.5 c.	3.5-4.5 c.	3.5-4.5 c.
Vegetables	1.5-2 c.	2-2.5 c.	2.5-3 c.	2.5-3 c.	3-3.5 c.	3.5-4.5 c.	4.5-5 c.	4.5-5 c.
Grains	5 oz-eq.	5-6 oz-eq.	6-7 oz-eq.	6-7 oz-eq.	7-8 oz-eq.	8-9 oz-eq.	9-10 oz-eq.	10-11 oz-eq.
Meat & Beans	4 oz-eq.	5 oz-eq.	5-5.5 oz-eq.	5.5-6.5 oz-eq.	6.5-7 oz-eq.	7-7.5 oz-eq.	7-7.5 oz-eq.	7.5-8 oz-eq.
Milk	2-3 c.	3 c.	3 c.	3 c.	3 c.	3 c.	3 c.	3 c.
Healthy Oils	4 tsp.	5 tsp.	5 tsp.	6 tsp.	6 tsp.	7 tsp.	8 tsp.	8 tsp.

Day/Date:

Breakfast: _____
Lunch: _____
Dinner: _____
Snacks: _____

GROUP	FRUITS	VEGETABLES	GRAINS	MEAT & BEANS	MILK	OILS
Goal Amount						
Estimate Your Total						
Total Calories						

Physical Activity: _____ Spiritual Activity: _____
Steps/Miles/Minutes: _____ My Emotions Today: ❑ Happy ❑ Sad ❑ Stressed

---

Day/Date:

Breakfast: _____
Lunch: _____
Dinner: _____
Snacks: _____

GROUP	FRUITS	VEGETABLES	GRAINS	MEAT & BEANS	MILK	OILS
Goal Amount						
Estimate Your Total						
Total Calories						

Physical Activity: _____ Spiritual Activity: _____
Steps/Miles/Minutes: _____ My Emotions Today: ❑ Happy ❑ Sad ❑ Stressed

---

Day/Date:

Breakfast: _____
Lunch: _____
Dinner: _____
Snacks: _____

GROUP	FRUITS	VEGETABLES	GRAINS	MEAT & BEANS	MILK	OILS
Goal Amount						
Estimate Your Total						
Total Calories						

Physical Activity: _____ Spiritual Activity: _____
Steps/Miles/Minutes: _____ My Emotions Today: ❑ Happy ❑ Sad ❑ Stressed

Copyright 2012 First Place 4 Health. Do not duplicate without permission from First Place 4 Health.

Day/Date: _____

Breakfast: _____
Lunch: _____
Dinner: _____
Snacks: _____

GROUP	FRUITS	VEGETABLES	GRAINS	MEAT & BEANS	MILK	OILS
Goal Amount						
Estimate Your Total						
Total Calories						

Physical Activity: _____ Spiritual Activity: _____
Steps/Miles/Minutes: _____ My Emotions Today: ❏ Happy ❏ Sad ❏ Stressed

---

Day/Date: _____

Breakfast: _____
Lunch: _____
Dinner: _____
Snacks: _____

GROUP	FRUITS	VEGETABLES	GRAINS	MEAT & BEANS	MILK	OILS
Goal Amount						
Estimate Your Total						
Total Calories						

Physical Activity: _____ Spiritual Activity: _____
Steps/Miles/Minutes: _____ My Emotions Today: ❏ Happy ❏ Sad ❏ Stressed

---

Day/Date: _____

Breakfast: _____
Lunch: _____
Dinner: _____
Snacks: _____

GROUP	FRUITS	VEGETABLES	GRAINS	MEAT & BEANS	MILK	OILS
Goal Amount						
Estimate Your Total						
Total Calories						

Physical Activity: _____ Spiritual Activity: _____
Steps/Miles/Minutes: _____ My Emotions Today: ❏ Happy ❏ Sad ❏ Stressed

---

Day/Date: _____

Breakfast: _____
Lunch: _____
Dinner: _____
Snacks: _____

GROUP	FRUITS	VEGETABLES	GRAINS	MEAT & BEANS	MILK	OILS
Goal Amount						
Estimate Your Total						
Total Calories						

Physical Activity: _____ Spiritual Activity: _____
Steps/Miles/Minutes: _____ My Emotions Today: ❏ Happy ❏ Sad ❏ Stressed

Live It Tracker

Name: _____ Date: _____ Week #: ____

Loss/gain ____ lbs. Calorie Range: _____ My food goal for the week: _____

Activity Level: None, < 30 min/day, 30-60 min/day, 60+ min/day My activity goal for the week: _____
My spiritual goal for the week: _____

Group	Daily Calories							
	1300-1400	1500-1600	1700-1800	1900-2000	2100-2200	2300-2400	2500-2600	2700-2800
Fruits	1.5-2 c.	1.5-2 c.	1.5-2 c.	2-2.5 c.	2-2.5 c.	2.5-3.5 c.	3.5-4.5 c.	3.5-4.5 c.
Vegetables	1.5-2 c.	2-2.5 c.	2.5-3 c.	2.5-3 c.	3-3.5 c.	3.5-4.5 c.	4.5-5 c.	4.5-5 c.
Grains	5 oz-eq.	5-6 oz-eq.	6-7 oz-eq.	6-7 oz-eq.	7-8 oz-eq.	8-9 oz-eq.	9-10 oz-eq.	10-11 oz-eq.
Meat & Beans	4 oz-eq.	5 oz-eq.	5-5.5 oz-eq.	5.5-6.5 oz-eq.	6.5-7 oz-eq.	7-7.5 oz-eq.	7-7.5 oz-eq.	7.5-8 oz-eq.
Milk	2-3 c.	3 c.	3 c.	3 c.	3 c.	3 c.	3 c.	3 c.
Healthy Oils	4 tsp.	5 tsp.	5 tsp.	6 tsp.	6 tsp.	7 tsp.	8 tsp.	8 tsp.

Day/Date:

Breakfast: _____
Lunch: _____
Dinner: _____
Snacks: _____

GROUP	FRUITS	VEGETABLES	GRAINS	MEAT & BEANS	MILK	OILS
Goal Amount						
Estimate Your Total						
Total Calories						

Physical Activity: _____ Spiritual Activity: _____
Steps/Miles/Minutes: _____ My Emotions Today: ❑ Happy ❑ Sad ❑ Stressed

Day/Date:

Breakfast: _____
Lunch: _____
Dinner: _____
Snacks: _____

GROUP	FRUITS	VEGETABLES	GRAINS	MEAT & BEANS	MILK	OILS
Goal Amount						
Estimate Your Total						
Total Calories						

Physical Activity: _____ Spiritual Activity: _____
Steps/Miles/Minutes: _____ My Emotions Today: ❑ Happy ❑ Sad ❑ Stressed

Day/Date:

Breakfast: _____
Lunch: _____
Dinner: _____
Snacks: _____

GROUP	FRUITS	VEGETABLES	GRAINS	MEAT & BEANS	MILK	OILS
Goal Amount						
Estimate Your Total						
Total Calories						

Physical Activity: _____ Spiritual Activity: _____
Steps/Miles/Minutes: _____ My Emotions Today: ❑ Happy ❑ Sad ❑ Stressed

Copyright 2012 First Place 4 Health. Do not duplicate without permission from First Place 4 Health.

Day/Date:

Breakfast: _____
Lunch: _____
Dinner: _____
Snacks: _____

GROUP	FRUITS	VEGETABLES	GRAINS	MEAT & BEANS	MILK	OILS
Goal Amount						
Estimate Your Total						
Total Calories						

Physical Activity: _____ Spiritual Activity: _____
Steps/Miles/Minutes: _____ My Emotions Today: ❏ Happy ❏ Sad ❏ Stressed

---

Day/Date:

Breakfast: _____
Lunch: _____
Dinner: _____
Snacks: _____

GROUP	FRUITS	VEGETABLES	GRAINS	MEAT & BEANS	MILK	OILS
Goal Amount						
Estimate Your Total						
Total Calories						

Physical Activity: _____ Spiritual Activity: _____
Steps/Miles/Minutes: _____ My Emotions Today: ❏ Happy ❏ Sad ❏ Stressed

---

Day/Date:

Breakfast: _____
Lunch: _____
Dinner: _____
Snacks: _____

GROUP	FRUITS	VEGETABLES	GRAINS	MEAT & BEANS	MILK	OILS
Goal Amount						
Estimate Your Total						
Total Calories						

Physical Activity: _____ Spiritual Activity: _____
Steps/Miles/Minutes: _____ My Emotions Today: ❏ Happy ❏ Sad ❏ Stressed

---

Day/Date:

Breakfast: _____
Lunch: _____
Dinner: _____
Snacks: _____

GROUP	FRUITS	VEGETABLES	GRAINS	MEAT & BEANS	MILK	OILS
Goal Amount						
Estimate Your Total						
Total Calories						

Physical Activity: _____ Spiritual Activity: _____
Steps/Miles/Minutes: _____ My Emotions Today: ❏ Happy ❏ Sad ❏ Stressed

Copyright 2012 First Place 4 Health. Do not duplicate without permission from First Place 4 Health.

let's count our miles!

Join the 100-Mile Club this Session

Can't walk that mile yet? Don't be discouraged! There are exercises you can do to strengthen your body and burn those extra calories. Keep a record on your Live It Tracker of the number of minutes you do these common physical activities, convert those minutes to miles following the chart below, and then mark off each mile you have completed on the chart found on the back of the back cover. Report your miles to your 100-Mile Club representative when you first arrive each week. Remember, you are not competing with anyone else . . . just yourself. Your job is to strive to reach 100 miles before the last meeting in this session. You can do it—just keep on moving!

Walking
slowly, 2 MPH	30 min.	= 156 cal.	= 1 mile
moderately, 3 MPH	20 min.	= 156 cal.	= 1 mile
very briskly, 4 MPH	15 min.	= 156 cal.	= 1 mile
speed walking	10 min.	= 156 cal.	= 1 mile
up stairs	13 min.	= 159 cal.	= 1 mile

Running/Jogging
	10 min.	= 156 cal.	= 1 mile

Cycling Outdoors
slowly, <10 MPH	20 min.	= 156 cal.	= 1 mile
light effort, 10-12 MPH	12 min.	= 156 cal.	= 1 mile
moderate effort, 12-14 MPH	10 min.	= 156 cal.	= 1 mile
vigorous effort, 14-16 MPH	7.5 min.	= 156 cal.	= 1 mile
very fast, 16-19 MPH	6.5 min.	= 152 cal.	= 1 mile

Sports Activities
Playing tennis (singles)	10 min.	= 156 cal.	= 1 mile
Swimming			
light to moderate effort	11 min.	= 152 cal.	= 1 mile
fast, vigorous effort	7.5 min.	= 156 cal.	= 1 mile
Softball	15 min.	= 156 cal.	= 1 mile
Golf	20 min.	= 156 cal	= 1 mile
Rollerblading	6.5 min.	= 152 cal.	= 1 mile
Ice skating	11 min.	= 152 cal.	= 1 mile

Jumping rope	7.5 min.	= 156 cal.	= 1 mile
Basketball	12 min.	= 156 cal.	= 1 mile
Soccer (casual)	15 min.	= 159 cal.	= 1 mile

Around the House

Mowing grass	22 min.	= 156 cal.	= 1 mile
Mopping, sweeping, vacuuming	19.5 min.	= 155 cal.	= 1 mile
Cooking	40 min.	= 160 cal.	= 1 mile
Gardening	19 min.	= 156 cal.	= 1 mile
Housework (general)	35 min.	= 156 cal.	= 1 mile
Ironing	45 min.	= 153 cal.	= 1 mile
Raking leaves	25 min.	= 150 cal.	= 1 mile
Washing car	23 min.	= 156 cal.	= 1 mile
Washing dishes	45 min.	= 153 cal.	= 1 mile

At the Gym

Stair machine	8.5 min.	= 155 cal.	= 1 mile
Stationary bike			
slowly, 10 MPH	30 min.	= 156 cal.	= 1 mile
moderately, 10-13 MPH	15 min.	= 156 cal.	= 1 mile
vigorously, 13-16 MPH	7.5 min.	= 156 cal.	= 1 mile
briskly, 16-19 MPH	6.5 min.	= 156 cal.	= 1 mile
Elliptical trainer	12 min.	= 156 cal.	= 1 mile
Weight machines (used vigorously)	13 min.	= 152 cal.	= 1 mile
Aerobics			
low impact	15 min.	= 156 cal.	= 1 mile
high impact	12 min.	= 156 cal.	= 1 mile
water	20 min.	= 156 cal.	= 1 mile
Pilates	15 min.	= 156 cal.	= 1 mile
Raquetball (casual)	15 min.	= 159 cal.	= 1 mile
Stretching exercises	25 min.	= 150 cal.	= 1 mile
Weight lifting (also works for weight machines used moderately or gently)	30 min.	= 156 cal.	= 1 mile

Family Leisure

Playing piano	37 min.	= 155 cal.	= 1 mile
Jumping rope	10 min.	= 152 cal.	= 1 mile
Skating (moderate)	20 min.	= 152 cal.	= 1 mile
Swimming			
moderate	17 min.	= 156 cal.	= 1 mile
vigorous	10 min.	= 148 cal.	= 1 mile
Table tennis	25 min.	= 150 cal.	= 1 mile
Walk/run/play with kids	25 min.	= 150 cal.	= 1 mile